Because You're Blind

REBECCA S MEADOWS

ISBN: 978-1-7349947-0-4 (Paperback)
ISBN: 978-1-7349947-1-1 (Kindle Mobi)
ISBN: 978-1-7349947-2-8 (ePub)
ISBN: 978-1-7349947-3-5 (Ingram)
ISBN: 978-1-7349947-4-2 (audible)

Published by BLUE BUTTERFLY ENTERPRISES, LLC

Contents

This book is dedicated to the staff at the Community Bridges Program, thank you for everything you have done for me.

It is dedicated to Robert M; I guess you were correct after all.

I would like to dedicate it to William G... wherever you are.

Most of all, I dedicate it to Phil McCready, with eternal gratitude for helping me get out of this nightmare that I found myself entangled in.

"And we know that in all things God works for the good of those who love Him, who have been called according to His purpose."

Romans 8:28
New International Version.

Acknowledgements

I want to thank my two sons for hugging Mommy when I really needed it. I want to thank all the people who have encouraged me over the years to tell my story. I want to say a special thanks to Darlene for her help locating the files. But most of all, I would like to thank my husband for his love and support during this project. He held me when I cried. He laughed with me when I had to find something to laugh about just so I wouldn't cry some more. He convinced me that my story is one that just had to be told but most of all he stood by me during those years when we were living through this epic nightmare together even though we didn't know how or if we would ever find our way out.

Introduction

$\mathcal{I}$ opened my eyes to find myself in darkness. I couldn't remember where I was or how I might have come to be there so I asked no one in particular "Where am I?"

A disembodied voice from somewhere in the darkness responded, "In the hospital." This made no sense to me. If I was in the hospital, why was it so dark? Hospitals are well lit places, right? So, I asked the next question.

"Why is it so dark?"

Again the voice responded, "Because you are blind."

It sounded so matter of fact, as if sudden blindness were a perfectly normal state to be in. I decided that it must be a dream (I had been experiencing some very strange dreams for a while and so this didn't surprise me in the least.) I simply closed my eyes and went back to sleep.

It was some time later when I again awoke and discovered to my horror that the blindness hadn't been a dream at all but an unspeakable real life event .

To this very day; nearly 30 years later,if I close my eyes, sometimes I still expect to wake up and find out I've been dreaming this whole time. Does that sound weird? I'm still asking myself in the back of my mind, "Why was I chosen to endure this life long and life-altering experience? I mean;why me out of all the souls that God created? Why did this happen to me? I remember being told the chance of this happening to me was something like one in a billion or something crazy like that. And then you have all the other unique and crazy things that have come as a result of this one in a billion lottery ticket I was handed when I was 12 years old. I also won the chance to be awarded a record settlement in the state of Montana. Then; years later, my rights and property were stripped from me in a most unprecedented plot in court that night in Havre and now; because of my strong feelings of being violated I'm writing what I hope will become an epic book with far reaching impacts on our society. I have actually changed the question I'm asking myself since I've been baptized in the Holy Spirit in December of 1998.It would take time for me to fully understand what had happened to cause this turn of events in my life. As the terror of this new reality engulfed me, I knew just one thing for certain; there was NO way I could live the rest of my life as a blind person.

The year was 1989. That year the Berlin Wall was torn down and "The Wind Beneath My Wings" sung by Bette Midler was a hit song. Bette Davis died that same year. It was the year that the state of Montana celebrated its centennial. In January of that year George Bush Sr. was sworn in as our 41st president.

I was a girl of 12 years old that summer when it all began. I awoke to the horror that would impact the rest of my life and would ultimately rob me of my personal freedom for almost 23 years. Waking up blind was a devastating reality for a child of 12 years old to come to terms with. I must tell you up front that my faith in God is the only thing that got me through those early years. This is my story.

Part One

What Came Before

Chapter One

I was raised in a lower middle-class family. My parents, my mother and stepfather, both worked really hard to support my three little sisters and me. They wanted to give us the upbringing they felt we deserved. My dad worked for the grain elevator loading box cars with grain brought into town by the local farmers. My mom cleaned houses for several people in town, both married couples and bachelors.

I remember when we were very small my mom would take my three little sisters and me to work with her. When I grew older we became latchkey kids. It was a very small town and definitely safe enough to do things like that. I remember how loved I felt back then. We all worked hard but we knew our parents loved us and would gladly die for us if they had the chance.

At times it was a difficult and harsh existence. I remember the climate being extremely dry and hot during the summers; it seemed as though we were always in a state of drought. In the fall, during harvest, dust clouds and tumble weeds were a hazard to small children. I remember countless grain trucks driving through the area, and my mother warning us about the danger when we went outside to play. In the fall, the colors were incredible. The sky was an endless blue, and there were golden wheat fields as far as the eye could see.

Winters were bitter cold with blowing snow and blizzards. Catching the bus to go to school meant walking to the highway. Our fingers and toes would ache from the freezing temperatures. I remember my stepdad stapling plastic over the windows to preserve heat. The wind was a mighty force that blew constantly.

This area was known as the Hi-Line, a group of small towns existing along U.S. Hi-Way 2 in north-central Montana. It was basically a small-town American farming community. It was a very safe place to raise children.

We lived in Hingham. My younger sisters and I attended Blue Sky School in Rudyard, a small town a few miles west of us.

I had always been called "bright" by my teachers and didn't have to make any effort to get excellent grades in school. I was active in girl scouts, drill team, girls' basketball and I also babysat for several families in our small community. I was an avid reader and my heart's desire was to grow up and become a teacher who could instill in children the same love of learning that I cherished.

This world I have just described was to come crashing down around my family in a nightmarish fashion. Our family has never fully recovered from what happened to us. This story is about what happened from my point of view.

Chapter Two

$\mathcal{I}$ was in the fourth grade when I began experiencing headaches. I continued having these headaches for over two years. There was no rhyme or reason to the timing of these episodes. Frequently I would awaken with them during the night. Other times I would wake up with them in the morning. Sometimes they would even come on later in the day. They always started small but grew in intensity until they felt like a huge bass drum was throbbing in my head. I would develop a horrible stomachache that would eventually result in violent vomiting. I always dreaded the inevitable point at which I would vomit but it would ease my stomach pain and my headache a bit so it was a real catch-22.

I remember laying there in bed as a child wondering if God was going to force me to spend the rest of my life like this. How did I anger Him enough to deserve this? I would learn much later that I had been dying at that time from something hidden in my brain.

I remember at night when I would wake up with one of my headaches and stumble to the bathroom to vomit. Often, I would collapse on the cold floor next to the toilet from exhaustion when I was done. I would lay there shivering with chills until I either passed out or regained my strength enough to find my way back to my bedroom. When I would awaken in the morning with one of these headaches, I could only lie there, dreading what I knew was coming. When I had them during the day at school I often felt like a freak, no one else I knew was going through this turmoil.

I also remember having headaches while I was in Minnesota visiting my dad and his family during the summers. I remember at least one occasion when I didn't make it to the bathroom to vomit and I accidentally got sick on my stepmother's floor. She became so angry at me. She screamed at me like a crazy lady. This treatment really frightened me; I was not accustomed to being screamed at when I was so ill.

One major trigger of my headaches seemed to be Big Lake. Each time my stepmother would take us swimming there I would experience one of my headaches. This was incredibly frustrating since it was one of my family's favorite places to go.

These episodes became so frequent that they almost seemed like a "normal" part of life. I continued experiencing these episodes until April of my sixth-grade year. It was then I experienced the final headache and my mom took me to see the doctor who had been "treating" me for migraines. I don't remember what happened after I fell asleep on the couch in the office at school waiting for my mom to come get me. The following information is based on what I was told by my family members after the fact.

My mom took me to Chester to see Dr. Andrews. When we arrived, after examining me, he and/or a colleague decided to transfer me to the hospital in Great Falls. They called an ambulance to come and transport me. The doctor instructed the ambulance crew that it was just a routine run, "Just take her to Great Falls and get her looked at to make sure she is alright." (No big deal). My mother rode in the ambulance with me. My stepfather followed in our family's old blue station wagon. My mother instructed the ambulance crew to go to Deaconess Hospital in Great Falls. As we entered the town I went into full arrest. When my dad saw the ambulance's lights and sirens come on he was relieved my mom was in the ambulance with me. He knew she would have been going nuts had she been in the car with him.

Upon arriving at the hospital, they were able to restart my heart and get me breathing again. It was at this time that a brain tumor was discovered and I was rushed into emergency surgery. When I came out of surgery, I lapsed into a coma.

That day, April 17, 1989, was the pivotal point when my life changed forever.

Part Two

The Dark Years

Chapter Three

When I awoke from my coma, as the following days turned into weeks, I slowly began to become more aware of what was going on in my environment. I learned that I had lapsed into a coma following the removal of a benign brain tumor that was the size of a lemon. It had been resting on my optic nerve and growing larger, presumably since I was born. I had remained in that deep comatose state for two and a half weeks following the procedure. As I slowly came out of the coma, there is a long period of time, several months in fact, where I do not remember much at all.

I was in a special bed that turned me regularly to prevent bed sores from developing while I was in my coma. My mom later told me it was a very expensive bed at the time. Clearly, the hospital spared no expense in making sure I had the best care available.

My days consisted of intensive therapy at the hands of the hospital staff who were diligently working to get my body and brain back into functioning order.

I found that I had suffered some fairly traumatic physical and mental damage.

I didn't fully comprehend at that point the extent of the damage or the full impact it would have on my future. At that point I thought the blindness was the worst of it. Boy, was I wrong!

While in the hospital I underwent intensive physical and occupational therapy to help me regain the function of the left side of my body. I had suffered paralysis and was weak from the time spent sleeping off my coma. That paralysis still affects me all these years later. It has been nearly 30 years since the experience but I still walk with a limp in my left leg. I also experience a slight tremor in my left hand on days when I am tired or not feeling well.

My circulation was also an issue. There were times my mom would comment that my legs were turning black because the blood wasn't making its way to my legs correctly. I couldn't see my legs turning black, but I did experience intense itching in my legs for a period of time until my circulation improved.

I was also put through very intensive speech therapy. This was not because of speech problems, rather it was to aid my brain in beginning to function properly again. I suffered horrible difficulties with cognitive functions because of the damage resulting from the pressure of the tumor on my brain. I couldn't manage the simplest of cognitive functions.

Becky H., my speech therapist (who we affectionately called "Big Becky" so there wouldn't be any confusion) administered aggressive therapy to assist my brain in beginning to function properly again.

I participated in these therapies for the term of my stay in the hospital. Even after I was eventually released my mother would transport me from our home in north central Montana back to Great Falls. I would take part in these treatments several times a week.

My family was instrumental in my early recovery. While I was still hospitalized they were right there beside me, encouraging me and not allowing me to give up. I became so tired and just wanted to quit. I could hardly handle the physical demand on my body and the pain in my muscles during the physical and occupational therapy. My mother, stepfather and little sisters encouraged me and pushed me to keep trying. We had all been raised to be hard workers so they knew I could do it but I know I would have given up had it not been for them.

My family and friends told me stories about things that happened during my early recovery while still in the hospital. I think my favorite story is the one my mom told me about how they kept a constant vigil at my bedside while I remained comatose. One day they saw me reaching up onto my face, fumbling around, searching for my nose. When I found it, I scratched it. This was the first sign of life in me since the surgery and they cheered.

That year for Mother's Day the gift my mother received was the hospital staff shut off my life support machines. This was a gift because it was at that point she finally knew I would survive without the assistance of machines.

Another story my mom told me was of one of the nurses whose care and professionalism stuck out in her mind. One day she came into my hospital room to find a gigantic burly man at my bedside. She noted how gentle and loving he was while taking care of her little girl. It turned out to be "Biker Mike", as he was known by his co-workers. Mike was a well-respected nurse with the hospital who rode his motorcycle into work every day.

Other stories that I remember were told to me by my best friend, Dawn. She told me she had read to me out of my favorite mystery series while I was sleeping. She knew I loved to read. My mom also told me a story about the Shriners coming to my hospital room to visit me (my grandma knew a bunch of them.) They came to my room dressed as clowns. My mom told me that they tied a helium filled, foil balloon to my bed. She said they knew I was aware something was there because I would attempt to strike at the balloon with my hand. Dawn also told me about doing the limbo while pushing me in my wheelchair at the hospital. It warms my heart even so many years later to think about the smiles my family and friends were able to enjoy during such a trying time.

I still remember how tired I would become during those therapy sessions. At the time I didn't foresee the reason for so much physical exertion. I didn't want to live anymore anyway. Thank God my family didn't give up on me.

I received counseling from a doctor in an effort to assist me in coping with the recent devastating changes in my life. At that point I was intensely focused on the blindness and the fact I no longer had any hope of fulfilling my dreams. I experienced very little benefit from these sessions. What could he say to make things better? He just couldn't change the blindness. The doctor eventually told my parents he no longer felt he could benefit me and at that point he was correct.

For a long time, I felt like I was having trouble breathing. It felt like a huge weight was resting on my chest. This was the extent of my grief. I cried myself to sleep every night, begging God to just kill me while I slept. I didn't want to live in this broken, useless body anymore.

I had to come to terms with my new reality on my own. It took a long time and much heartache before I could live without the suffocating grief that engulfed me each day.

During this time I felt so alone. God was the only one I could cry out to. Even after I started regaining some light perception and blurry vision, my life didn't get any better. I had simply gone to sleep on the couch at school like I had done so many times before. I then awoke to find myself trapped in a profoundly dark and frightening alternate reality. It was like falling through the rabbit hole into a nightmarish Wonderland.

My mom was unable to comprehend my deep level of despair. Counseling had been unsuccessful in alleviating my anguish. I felt like no one understood what I was going through. In an attempt to help me deal with the distress and shock of the situation, medication was prescribed.

I remained on several medications when I returned home from the hospital. One of them was Lithium. They put me on this medication in an effort to control my depression and mood swings. This was a bad decision. I was not depressed because of a chemical imbalance in my brain that could be corrected with the introduction of synthetic chemicals; The situation I found myself in was what caused my misery. I was very discouraged and unhappy due to the turn my life had taken. When I was on Lithium I still felt deep sorrow and grief. Handling my day to day life was so much worse on the drug because I had to keep the feelings bottled up inside; I couldn't express them. I think a better way to help someone in this situation would be to teach them how to communicate their feelings, not cover them up with drugs.

As a result of being on the wrong medication, I began to have suicidal thoughts. When I began to have these thoughts I decided to stockpile my Lithium, planning on overdosing on it when I had several pills at once. After I had been off the drug for a while I stopped having those dangerous ideas, so I simply flushed the pills down the toilet.

During this time my mom was taking me back to Great Falls several times a week. I had medical checkups and continuing therapy sessions. There was always a blood test. The doctors were continually tracking factors related to my brain and body. One of their concerns was my Lithium level. Realizing that I couldn't hide my secret any longer, I confessed to my mom that I had stopped taking the drug. She called the doctor right away and told him that I had been off my medication for some time. He said that since I had been doing fine without it not to worry.

The doctors also had me on anti-seizure medication. I had experienced Grand Mal seizures when they relieved the pressure from my brain.

They had also given me steroids while I was in the hospital to make my body stronger and help me survive what was happening to me. To this day I still suffer the effects of those steroids; growing hair in places it is not normal for a woman to have hair. I also develop muscle tone on my body with very little effort. My first child was abnormally large; he was the second largest baby ever born here at the hospital. My second son was also larger than average. I can't help but wonder how much of this can be attributed to those steroids.

Another reason for continued tracking of the condition of my blood was my white blood cell count. Whether it was another result of the brain injury or simply a side-effect of the medications; my white count dropped dramatically. It was so low that the doctors were very concerned about my health. Over time they continued monitoring it. They noticed that when I would get sick my white count would come up and fight off the illness. The doctors eventually decided it was alright.

My hair was also impacted negatively by the surgery and subsequent drugs they had me on. It had always been naturally curly prior to the brain tumor but now it was very unmanageable. I remember my mom getting so cross when she would try to curl it. These locks wouldn't hold a curl and when she would take me to get a perm my hair would only burn and wind up in worse condition. My hair remained unmanageable until 1998 when I shaved my head completely bald and started over with a new do. It is much more manageable now.

I remember one day when my parents received an emergency call from Dr. H., my blood doctor. We had gone to Great Falls that day and they had drawn my blood. As it turned out my seizure medication had dropped drastically and he was concerned about my safety. My parents immediately rushed me back to the hospital. The medical staff eventually decided the seizure medication was no longer a necessity and they stopped prescribing it.

My mom spent countless hours on the road driving me back and forth for medical appointments. She was so fatigued that she actually fell asleep at the wheel one night as we were returning home. Miraculously, she awoke when the car hit the rumble strips on the edge of the highway. We were crossing the span between Great Falls and Chester via the "Chester cut across" (as it was known by locals.) It was a road that people took off the beaten path to make the trip between Great Falls and Chester shorter. My parents always used it. Our home was about an hour and a half north of Great Falls so there was a lot of driving. I remember the motor blew out of my parents' old blue station wagon from all those trips.

In the midst of my therapy, my mom took me to the deaf and blind school in Great Falls for the summer orientation program. At the school they tried to force me to learn braille. This proved impossible however. The feeling in my fingertips was almost nonexistent and I had such short term memory loss, it was impossible for me to remember what those little dots meant, if I managed to feel them at all. I kept insisting that I knew God wasn't going to leave me totally blind, He wouldn't do that to me. They told me that I couldn't count on that. I guess He proved them wrong.

Chapter Four

Once I was at home again and things returned to normal (if you can call it that) I was sent back to school with my sisters in the fall. Because of the brain tumor, the decision was made that I should be held back a year. Therefore, I began the year in Mr. M.'s sixth grade class again. There was one good thing about this decision. The school permitted me to stay home on days when I was just too tired. My brain and body were exerting a lot of energy in those early days; not only to start the healing process but also to grow. I was, after all, just entering adolescence. Since I had already technically passed sixth grade, the school was more lenient with me about how many days I missed.

Mr. M.'s face is the last one I recall seeing clearly before I went blind. I remember the last day of school when I had the final headache. He had taken me to the school office so I could rest on the couch. I waited for my mom to arrive at the school, pick me up, and take me to the doctor. This had been the regular routine when I would have one of my headaches at school. I remember looking up at him while he ran copies at the copy machine. Mr. M. had been my coach for girls' basketball that year. He was a great teacher and coach who genuinely cared about his students. He inquired if I would be alright. Little did I know as I closed my eyes, the next time I opened them it would be as a totally different person.

In the fall of 1989, as I entered Mr. M.'s class for a second time, I was placed in my little sister's class. This became a symbol of great shame for me. I had been a very intelligent young lady, not someone who was held back in school.

That year the school hired Mary, a woman from the community, to be my aide in class. She read my books to me and wrote things down for me. I remember she was pregnant so it turned out to be a good job for her.

I was the first severely handicapped student Blue Sky had ever mainstreamed into the student body. The school really bent over backwards to accommodate me. In addition to hiring Mary I was provided with a talking calculator to use for math.

The first year back at Blue Sky was very difficult for me. I was grieving the sudden loss of my sight. I didn't even realize that I had a severe brain injury to go along with the blindness. My social skills were horrible. My peers were just entering adolescence themselves so they were unable to show me any empathy.

I remember one outing with my best friend Dawn during those early days. We went to the mall in Havre. She was so uncomfortable with me; she wouldn't even sight guide me. Her idea was that we would walk through the mall and occasionally bump arms to enable me to know my way. This did not work of course and I insisted she sight guide me. She was concerned that people would think she was "gay" if I held onto her arm. At the time I just blew off her concerns. I was blind and she was my friend. She should sight guide me. Now, as an adult, I understand what she was going through. She didn't understand what had happened to me any better than I did. No adult was counseling us on any of it. The situation was horrible. My sisters, close friends, and I; none of us understood what was happening. We were only children at the time. I was living in the darkest part of it; all alone.

For the entire time I went to Blue Sky after the tumor, when I would pass Dawn in the halls, I was very sad. I didn't know how to reach out to this girl who had once been my best friend. It was incredibly lonely for me and I found out years later when we were grown that Dawn had been going through the same feelings.

There were many difficult experiences that resulted from the brain tumor. These situations affected everyone around me. My family at home was impacted financially as well as emotionally.

At the time I fell ill I was covered by my biological father's medical insurance through his job in Plymouth, Minnesota. My stepdad's insurance was a secondary guarantor for my coverage.

My biological dad's insurance refused to pay my bills at one point because according to them the brain tumor had been a "preexisting condition." My parents battled with the insurance company for a long time to get the bills paid.

During this time I remember feeling a strong sense of guilt because of what was happening to my family. I was the one who had fallen ill. Was my life really worth all the horrible experiences my family was having?

I was a child at the time and had so much on my plate. While everyone around me was falling apart in their own way, I was dealing with much larger issues. Not only was I dealing with guilt, I was still trying to get a grip on my new situation. How was I going to overcome my blindness and ever be able to live a complete and normal life? I was also trying to figure out how to help my mother and sisters through their emotional turmoil. My stepdad was our rock. Each member of my family seemed to be impacted by the traumatic situation in different ways. Being so young, I was only able to deal with my own issues. Everyone else's trauma was a separate entity that only added to my burden.

My mom was heartbroken watching her little girl go through this hell but she didn't know how to comfort me. When I would cry from the grief she would simply yell at me, "You might as well stop bawling because there is nothing you can do about it anyway!" My stepdad on the other hand would hold me and allow me to cry out my pain and hopelessness. It would be a long time before my mom finally reached the point where she was able to allow herself to cry out her pain also. Maybe she cried in private back then, never where I could hear her. When she finally did cry with me I could feel her tears on my head and back as she held me and we cried together. Crying may not be cool but there are times in life when you must or you will crack up. This was our private hell.

There was a huge amount of stress in our house, especially between my mom and me. We exchanged a lot of hurtful words during those early years. One time she even became aggressive with me. At the time we were yelling at each other and I, at least, was crying. She finally lost it.

Life went on like this for a long time. I don't even know what my little sisters were feeling back then. They had watched their big sister go from a vibrant, healthy young girl with all the potential in the world to a shell of a girl who was barely clinging to sanity and our mom was losing it also. I think it was our dad who held it all together. I later discovered we were unraveling at some level that remained unseen. My mother lost her commitment to our family.

Ami has shared with me how she felt when she was a child and became a care giver to her older sister. It was a role reversal. I became as a small child in need of intensive care and my little sister Ami was forced to be that care giver. As the oldest, I had always looked after and protected my little sisters. Now the situation had changed. I believe this reversal in the natural order greatly affected Ami. The frustration of my helplessness was overwhelming. I was expected to obey everyone, even my little sisters. It was quite humiliating. My parents didn't seem to care about or be aware of what their daughters were going through.

Because of everything that transpired, our family has been shattered. Today, nearly thirty years later, we don't speak to each other. My sister Ami is the only one of my family members who I have spoken to in several years. Even when I did have any contact with the rest of the family, it was always a negative experience. I think they harbor ill feelings toward me because of what happened.

I know my mom blamed herself for a long time for not taking me to a different doctor, but what can a person expect of themselves? I have never held her responsible for the brain tumor.

Hindsight is 20/20. Today I can honestly say that I can see how God worked it all together for my good. I just wish the rest of my family was dealing with it as well as I am.

Another memory I have is of my little sister, Lynn. She was having nightmares. My mom would discover her sleep walking outside her bedroom door with her eyes wild. She would tell my mom, "The house is on fire! I have to get Becky out!" When my mom would tell our family at the breakfast table about finding Lynn like this the night before, I was terribly sad. Clearly my little sister was so traumatized she was having nightmares.

Lynn was very sensitive. She was always protective of her sisters. I recall one occasion when we were little girls before the tumor when Ami, Lynn and I were walking around town. Steve, an older kid who lived in our town and owned a motorcycle was chasing us around while riding his bike. He would often find us out on the streets and engage in this behavior. It terrified us horribly but now, looking back as an adult, I suspect he was just incredibly bored in Hingham and found it great fun to torment us this way. He never actually hit one of us on his motorcycle and I am sure he could have had he really wanted to.

On this particular occasion, he had trapped us on a dead end street. We huddled together to discuss how we would get out of this fix. While we were discussing it, Lynn announced that she would run in another direction, causing Steve to follow her so we could escape. Ami and I were horrified at the prospect of our little sister sacrificing herself in this manner so we said, "No!"

This did not dissuade Lynn. She took off running. I was mortified. How could I allow my little sister to sacrifice herself in this manner? Steve let us go and all worked out but it was a good example of how Lynn felt about her sisters.

Steve was always a trouble maker. He broke into several buildings in our town. One time he stole a gun from my stepdad. On another occasion he stood up on the roof of the old school in Hingham and shot at my little sisters with a bow and arrows. Like I said, I think he was really bored. He found ways to amuse himself.

One summer when I was a kid, I was away in Minnesota visiting my biological father. Steve found my sister Ami out alone and he attacked her, raping her. It was years later, after we became adults, before I learned of this incident. My friend Polly witnessed the rape from afar. She could hear Ami screaming. Polly knew what was happening to my little sister because Steve had done the same to her. She had warned Ami not to go with him into the Quonset hut where the rape occurred. Polly went with Ami to my parents and told them what had transpired with Steve. My parents refused to get any help for Ami or press charges against Steve. I believe this contributed to my sister's problems later in life.

My sister Ami has had many struggles as an adult. I believe many of these problems can be traced back to the abuse and neglect we suffered at the hands of our parents. My parents always had a flippant attitude about our health and safety when we were children. Ami was cursed with horrible ear infections when we were little. My parents didn't get her decent medical care and her ear drum wound up rupturing.

Our dad's typical reaction when we would complain about any physical malady was, "Come out to the garage and I will cut it off with the chain saw." He was only kidding but they didn't take us to doctors. I was fortunate to see Dr. Andrews when I was a kid. We were taught that pain was a part of life and we better learn to deal with it. This notion works sometimes but when major medical problems come up, you need a doctor.

As a result of everything that occurred, Ami really doesn't have any relationship with our parents. Then again, neither do I.

Several years ago, I was discussing this situation with our sister Jo. She still has a close relationship with our parents. She told me that our mom acts as though Ami and I are dead. I suspect Joanne, our mother, views us as some kind of blemish on her record. We are her two big mistakes. I am, in her mind, damaged and no longer good enough for her. Ami has chosen an alternative lifestyle and my mother just can't stand that. Knowing my mother, I suspect she is very embarrassed to have , people looking down at her because of us. She thinks that if she pretends we are dead, maybe we will be. I guess she got what she wanted. I will not allow her around my family because she is not a well person.

I have struggled for many years to understand why my mom doesn't want to know me anymore. It is as if she would rather remember the damaged little girl I was after the tumor. She doesn't care to know me now that I have recovered from what happened to me. I wonder if part of this is due to the fact that if she acknowledges that I am a more or less whole and complete person in spite of what happened; she would have to admit that what she did to me was scandalous and unnecessary. Although I have recovered, there has been a great deal of loss. Unfortunately, a person just can't turn back the clock.

Chapter Five

or years after the tumor I struggled to understand how my brain could betray me. That is just what it felt like; a betrayal from within.

It was terribly difficult, who could you blame? God? Tried that, but I knew He loved me. My mom? Tried that also but it didn't feel right either. She was so destroyed by what had happened. *She* ultimately blamed the doctor.

It was during the first year back at school that my mom came to me and suggested she could file a lawsuit against Dr. Andrews on my behalf. Apparently someone had suggested this to her. I agreed; wanting something, *anything* to make things better. We had always been poor, perhaps money was the answer.

She sought out an attorney and filed her lawsuit. It was a medical malpractice lawsuit. As it turned out, she didn't sue the doctor. He worked for the federal government so she wound up suing the feds. This is when her focus changed from what was best for me to the money she could get.

Honestly, I think initially she did want to do what was best for me. Just as I had thought that maybe money could make things better, she realized it did make things better—for *her.*

She found a good attorney. He knew how to sue the government. He knew how to win.

Several things happened to prepare for the lawsuit. My medical records were pulled together. I was put in the hospital in Missoula for

24

a week long evaluation. A team of doctors and therapists examined me to determine the extent of damage to my brain and body. They also predicted how my various injuries might impact the rest of my life. I was told my teacher at Blue Sky also agreed to testify in court if need be. I feel Mr. M's testimony would have been quite significant because he had been my basketball coach as well as my classroom teacher both before and just after the tumor so I'm sure he had a good picture of how the tumor had impacted me. I remember being told all the information that was gathered would be set before a medical board. The board would then determine an approximate dollar value for what they supposed my future costs would be. These experts predicted a life expectancy for me. They needed to figure out how much money the lawsuit was worth. It's hard to imagine how someone could even think of putting a dollar value on a person's life, especially a child's.

The preparation for the lawsuit was done and my life went on.

During this time, kids I had known for years and grown up with would approach me at school and ask, "Is it true you are going to get (_) dollars?" It was always a different dollar amount. That is how rumors work. They change a little bit each time they are repeated and in this case the dollar amount always grew exponentially. The gossip drove an even wider wedge between my peers and me. Everyone's parents worked labor intensive jobs. What entitled *my* family to all of this money?

I was told at home not to talk about the lawsuit or money with anyone. My mom, however, was apparently telling all her friends because it was getting around the community somehow. *I* was instructed not to say a word to anyone , but I overheard my mother gossiping with many people. Sure, my little sisters could have been talking but I seriously doubted if they knew any more information than I did.

It was incredibly frustrating when I was confronted at school by my peers in this fashion. What was I supposed to say? I had been told nothing and was instructed not to say a word. The kids seemed to think I was keeping something from them. I am not a liar so I couldn't just make something up.

occasionally, my mother's lawyers would come to our home and take her away to some unknown location. They would meet with the lawyers from the government to negotiate the lawsuit. When she returned from one of these meetings she announced to me that she had settled the suit. The dollar amount really didn't mean anything to me at that point. How could any amount of money heal the wounds our family had sustained due to what happened? She, however, was very excited about it all.

I was astounded. How had she managed to get so much money from the government when I was the one who had become sick? I had never even spoken to one of the lawyers for the government.

The lawsuit was settled out of court in 1992. My mother also received a substantial settlement for *her* suffering.

It was really embarrassing how fast my parents walked through the money. From rags to riches and back again!

The amount of money my mother wound up settling for on my behalf was substantially less than the medical board had calculated for the lawsuit. The theory was, however, if the money was invested wisely, it would sustain me. It was like playing Russian Roulette with my future.

After the lawsuit was settled a firm in Great Falls was hired to invest my funds. My mother had herself appointed as my conservator so she could "manage" my assets.

It was after the lawsuit was settled that my mom began collecting a paycheck from my account. Her reasoning was interesting. She justified the check by claiming that she quit her job to "take care of me." The funny thing was, after she was home for a while she got bored. She went back to work and left me at home alone while continuing to collect the paycheck from my account. Like I said, she knew how the money could benefit her. She also would occasionally present me with various purchases she had decided to buy with my money. She always had a justification. Usually it was something for her or my little sisters that I "owed" them because it was so horrible living with me. It was always impressed upon me that I had to be careful on how I spent my money, because it had to last me for the rest of my life. My mother did not appear to be constrained by the same ideals. She also impressed upon me that she and my dad had spent my sisters' college funds to get by when times were tough following the tumor incident. I also owed them because of that. There was never any mention of what had happened to *my* college fund, if there had ever been one. I think this was another lie from my mom to manipulate me. When she would present me with purchases she thought I "owed" her or my sisters, if I didn't readily agree to the purchase she would accuse me of being "greedy." To this day I don't know why she ever bothered to ask me my opinion. It wasn't as if I could do anything to stop her from buying whatever she wanted. I literally was not allowed to make any decisions on how *my* money would be spent.

I had no allies. There was no one overseeing my mother's activities except for a judge in Havre who would occasionally see her in court. He believed whatever she told him. It was truly comical listening to my mom when she would find out that the judge wanted to see her. She was always nervous. If the judge found out what really had been going on with my funds, she would have been in big trouble. My mother would tell me things like "You know you owe this to us because..." and then would add whatever her excuse was at the time, like I was the one who was going to be holding her accountable, not the judge. I felt like she was threatening me because she actually thought the judge may ask me what had been going on, but he never spoke to me. Sometimes she would be furious with me when she would discuss the fact that I "owed this to them". She was put in the position where she had been enabled to misuse my funds. It was as if it was my fault because if it hadn't been for me, she wouldn't have been put in this situation to begin with. I was very scared being put in this position. My mother definitely had a guilty conscience but only she could change her behavior.

One day there was a stranger in Hingham putting signs up for the judge's reelection campaign. My mom told me that if he approached me to talk to me I was not to speak to him. She was afraid the judge may have asked the man to see if he could find out anything regarding my situation while he was in town. She thought the man may have been the judge's son. I was really confused when she told me not to talk to the man if he approached me. How do you not speak to someone without being rude?

Chapter Six

After the first year at Blue Sky my parents opted to send me to the Montana School for the Deaf and Blind in Great Falls (MSDB). I lived in a dorm at the school. On the weekends my parents would come and pick me up in Great Falls or I would take the Greyhound bus to Havre to reduce their drive. The state paid for students to go home one weekend a month to see their families.

I was somewhat happy at MSDB because at least I had friends and the facility was designed for blind people. At MSDB I received a white cane and was given mobility training. I went to MSDB for that entire school year and part of the following.

I remember at MSDB when the other students and I would hang out together. We sat together at lunch and visited. On other occasions we walked around campus together. It was so nice having friends again. Some of the staff members were also disabled so they understood a lot of what we were going through.

Things were so bad at home that I began trying to stay at MSDB whenever I could. On the weekend that the state paid for students to go home, I had to leave. When my mom would want me to come home on extra weekends, however, I would try to get out of it. I really felt like my mom only wanted me for her own financial gain. I didn't understand why she wanted me home so badly. The lawsuit hadn't been settled yet at that point so it didn't really matter if she was "taking care" of me. I guess maybe she had some kind of need to have me near her although I can't imagine why-we didn't get along. I think perhaps she was trying to make our situation "appear" to be one where she was concerned for me. Maybe her attorneys told her that it was better for the lawsuit if she was "taking care" of me and therefore deserved some kind of reimbursement for her trouble.

My home life was horrible. The cloud of depression that permeated our home was overwhelming. Life at home was very frustrating for me. My family made no effort to make the living environment safe for me. I would stumble around the house knocking things over. My mom was constantly cross with me because of the messes I made. I even fell down the basement stairs at times. Our stairs were old wooden steps and very steep.

On one occasion my parents took my little sisters and me camping with some of their friends. I tripped on a tent stake and tore the tent of my mother's friend. My mother was furious with me but what was I supposed to do? She would not give me a white cane and I was blind.

One year my parents took us on a trip for Christmas. On the trip they rented snowmobiles. I was leery of riding on the machines because I couldn't see. My parents forced me to get on with my sister Ami driving. My sister was a dare devil and she drove like a nut. I was scared stiff! I couldn't see where we were going and it felt as if I would fall off at any moment. Again, my parents didn't care about what I was feeling. I was pleading with my sister to slow down, to stop going over the jumps so fast. Rather, Ami continued her out of control driving. She finally stopped and took my helmet off. It was then she realized how petrified I was and regretted ignoring my pleas. She had thought I was kidding. I then climbed on the snowmobile that Lynn was driving. Lynn was much more conscious of my fears. It was a much better experience after that.

Chapter Seven

In the second year I was at MSDB, I fell and dislocated my shoulder. My mother took me home for the recovery period. I was supposed to wear my sling on my arm for six weeks to ensure my shoulder had time to heal properly. I had been home for less than two weeks when my mom took my sling away and sent me back to school at Blue Sky.

I am not sure why she made these decisions. They seemed irresponsible and senseless. My dislocated shoulder had not yet healed. She also removed me, a blind girl, from a blind school and stuck me in a public school that was ill equipped to accommodate my needs. It was detrimental to my peace of mind and my functionality in a school setting. As a result of this poor decision, I struggled to complete my high school education.

Since my shoulder didn't heal properly, I still experience great amounts of pain in it to this day.

When I was at MSDB I also went to the Deaconess Hospital in the cab for continuing speech therapy several times a week. This also came to an abrupt halt after my mom pulled me out of MSDB.

When my mom sent me back to public school I had no one-on-one assistance. She was embarrassed by my blindness and refused to allow me to use my cane at school. I remember several times when I fell down the stairs in the school building. Struggling to get through the crowd of students to make it to class on time proved to be impossible. Several of the teachers were pretty tough on me initially because I was always late for class. Over time they eventually stopped badgering me about my lack of punctuality. I'm not sure if they just gave up trying to correct my tardiness or if they realized the difficulties I experienced while navigating the halls.

When I was sent back to public school I was told that the curriculum I had been taught at MSDB had included seventh and eighth grade material. This meant I had "completed" both grades while I was there. I never bought this. My mom had a habit of telling lies just to accomplish her agenda. I think my mom wanted me back where I belonged.

As I continued at Blue Sky things never became easier for me. One day I was actually assaulted in the hallway.

The school dealt with the situation the best they could; but what could be done? I was a blind victim who was assaulted from behind, making it impossible for me to defend myself. My mother ultimately told me that it was my fault I had been assaulted. I was bent over, digging through books on the floor of my locker, when someone began massaging my vaginal area. He made some really crude comments while doing so. I felt filthy and violated when this was done to me. When the school did their investigation, there were no other witnesses, even though the bell had rung and the halls were swarming with students making their way to the next class.

Despite all the horrible experiences, there was one good thing I took from my years at Blue Sky. I learned word processing. I am very comfortable on a computer keyboard and can type without struggling to see the keys.

After that first year back at Blue Sky when I was confronted with numerous challenges, the decision was made that I should spend the majority of my time in the special education room. It was my sophomore year.

The special education teacher, Mrs. Matt, and I got along extremely well. We saw differently on social issues but she was good at her job and I was very comfortable in her classroom. I still didn't have any friends though. It was a lonely existence.

One of the activities the students in Mrs. Matt's room participated in was taking care of the pop and juice machines in the hallway. On Fridays we would restock the machines with beverages. We would then roll the change and count the dollar bills. The money was prepared to be deposited in the bank. Some of us also completed a form showing what pop and juice we needed to order from the distributor when he returned.

I became friends with Polly in Mrs. Matt's classroom. I had known Polly since I was very young. She had always been an outcast among the other students but once we had the chance to get to know each other we became fast friends.

It was Polly who led me to the Lord during this time. She shared her faith with me. I had always felt drawn to the Lord so I prayed. I knew He was there for me when times were tough.

It was more than just a feeling that started after the brain tumor. My parents would take us four girls to the Lutheran church in our town when I was little. They never demonstrated faith themselves; it was just something they felt obligated to do because all respectable parents in our little community took their kids to church.

I was the only one of my mom's children who really wanted to go. When we would go to church I loved listening to the pastor preach out of the scriptures and the Bible stories our Sunday school teacher would tell. I hungered for more of God. Like I said, I had always known God was out there calling me. I have a strong belief that God calls all of us; if only we would listen.

Polly had grown up in a family that was in a financial bracket just below mine. Economically, she was the poorest student at school. I dwell on our respective economic statuses only to impress upon the reader what the situation was. In our school if your family was "low-income" you were not accepted. It was just a fact of life we grew up understanding. Polly's mother died of cancer when she was very young. Her dad was an alcoholic. The kids at school would taunt her mercilessly when we were in elementary school. When I was little, I tried taking part in teasing her one time. It made me feel sick to engage in such cruel behavior, though. I never did it again.

During those years when I was dealing with my condition and the resulting grief, Polly had been going through some pretty horrible circumstances herself. She had slit her wrists and spent time in recovery. I am not completely clear on everything she went through but I understand it was an awful experience for her.

Polly and I remained friends for the rest of our time at Blue Sky.

Polly was a year ahead of me. She graduated the year before I did. Prior to her graduation, we were always together. We spent so much time together that when fellow students would see me without her they would inquire where she was. It was enriching to have someone to hang out and eat lunch with. During my senior year, after Polly was gone, I was terribly lonely once again.

We remain friends today. She is my only real friend from high school. I take my two sons to where she lives several times a year so my children and hers can play together. It is a good opportunity for us to catch up and spend time together.

It was during those early years that my dad lost his job at the grain elevator. It was explained to me that the Japanese had bought the elevator and fired my dad's boss and the only other employee who worked there. Apparently they just kept my dad on to finish loading the last train. Then they would fire him as well. This made my dad sore so he just quit.

After my dad quit his job at the grain elevator he went to work at the nursing home in Chester as a custodian. My mother had already been working there as a CNA. All three of my little sisters also went to work there when they turned fifteen.

This was very hard for me, watching my whole family work. All I could do was sit at home alone. I longed to go to work also. Alas; this was not possible back then.

During those early years I came face to face with Dr. Andrews. I was sick and my mother took me up to the clinic in Chester to see Dr. Ross.

He was my pediatrician from Great Falls, and also worked at the clinic in Chester part time. (I think this was something doctors did at that time in an effort to provide better medical care to people on the Hi-Line.)

While we were at the clinic we were approached by someone. Of course I couldn't see the person so when the man spoke to me directly, addressing me by name, I assumed he was Dr. Ross. When I responded to him, calling him "Dr. Ross" the man quietly denied the association. I was confused. My mother angrily ordered the man to tell me who he was. He then revealed to me that he was Dr. Andrews.

This shocked me. Since the tumor incident my mother had been very verbal about her feelings regarding Dr. Andrews. She harbored great anger and hostility toward him for what had happened. I remember my mother talking about a strong desire to gouge out Dr. Andrews eyes. Her rage greatly frightened me. I had not yet come to terms with my feelings regarding him. At that point I was still grappling with blaming God. This is my first recollection of having seen Dr. Andrews since that day in April of 1989, when circumstances went so terribly wrong. I haven't come into contact with him since.

I don't think I have ever really "blamed" Dr. Andrews for what happened. It was just an error in judgment that happened to cause me a great deal of suffering and has significantly impacted my life. Who can say why it happened? Only God knows why He permitted it.

After this incident we were told by Joanne's lawyers that Dr. Andrews had admitted his fault so we no longer needed to prove he had erred in his treatment of me. I think that he just needed to see for himself the consequences of what had transpired on that April day.

Chapter Eight

I have had many unusual feelings and experiences that resulted from my brain injury. I want to describe some of these in an effort to help people better understand what a person experiences when living with a brain injury.

One devastating consequence that resulted from the brain injury was amnesia. I have always remembered names of people and places but have no real memory of specific events that occurred before the tumor incident. For example, when my friends would talk about specific ball games we had played in or birthday parties and the like, I couldn't remember them. I had lost these cherished childhood events forever. I knew they had happened only because my friends were describing them to me. There was a keen sense of having been truly happy back then although I lost all memory of why my life was so carefree. I have never regained those lost memories.

When I initially awoke from my coma the personnel at the hospital had asked me questions to test my memory. They asked me how old I was. I responded by saying eleven years old. I had forgotten my twelfth birthday. They also asked me who the president was. I replied Ronald Reagan, having forgotten the fact that a new president had been elected a few months earlier.

I don't remember what other questions they asked but they were able to develop an idea of how severe my memory loss was.

Understandably, I also experienced great difficulty accepting my sudden blindness. I couldn't foresee a day when things might get better.

Some of this was no doubt due to my tender age. Falling asleep and then waking up in this new and life-shattering circumstance was such a shock to my young mind and spirit, it was nearly more than I could bear.

For several years after the incident I suffered from insomnia. I was exhausted when I would go to bed. Initially, sleep would come quite quickly but I would awaken in the middle of the night. My mind would be racing through various thoughts. I couldn't make my brain slow down and was unable to return to sleep. This went on virtually every night. Eventually I discovered that concentrating on my breathing helped. Focusing on my inhales and exhales would get the focus off of my racing thoughts and force my brain to slow down. This would work for a while until my mind would wander away, back to the racing thoughts.

There were times when I would awaken and not know where I was. I would lay there awake struggling to remember where I had been when I lay down to go to sleep. I didn't often sleep away from home but I still experienced this frequently.

There were nights when I would wake up and have to go to the bathroom. I would stand up quickly and begin to seek it out. After I was out in the large, open room in my parent's basement that lay between my bedroom and the bathroom, it was as if I would become completely awake. I would find that I was disoriented, like my brain had not been fully conscious when I had first gotten out of bed. Then at that moment I would wake up the rest of the way. This created a problem for me. Because it was so dark in the basement, I would have to try to get my bearings so I could set out once again for the bathroom. For example, I would "wake up" at the foot of the stairs near my Dad's hunting room or back behind the furnace near where my sister Ami slept. I would have to stay calm and try to remember what the basement looked like. Where was the bathroom in relation to where I found myself?

Often, by the time I found the bathroom, I was afraid I would wet myself I had to go so bad. That is how long I would wander around the basement trying to find my way. I also experienced this in hotels and at the homes of other family members when I would sleep there.

Every morning when I woke up I didn't know what day it was; even what month or year. I began spending time lying in bed when I woke up trying to remember the date, what I had done the day before, and what was on the agenda for that day. It would take me a long time to finally recall the information, if I managed to retrieve it at all. It really seemed like my brain had trouble waking up all the way.

I remember a particular occasion when this happened to me. This incident occurred when I was still living with my mom after I graduated from high school. One morning I awoke disoriented and confused. I thought I was late for school. In a panic, I rushed upstairs and told my mom that I was late for school and needed to hurry. She just sat there, offering no help. She calmly told me that I didn't go to school. This made me even more frantic. I thought she was only trying to put me off; that she was trying to prevent me from getting an education in order to keep me under her control. After all, she had always done that anyway. I had completely forgotten that I had graduated from high school. Once again, my brain hadn't quite woken up all the way to process my environment correctly. Throughout the time when my brain was having so much trouble with these minor tasks; I was, of course, unable to retain information I was learning at school.

For years following the tumor I felt somewhat separated from the rest of my person. My brain felt different, as if it wasn't connected to me completely. It didn't process thoughts the way it should. When I would attempt to dwell on anything I couldn't pull off a complete sequence of thoughts without getting distracted and my mind wandering off in a thousand different directions.

I was told the reason I couldn't see was because my brain wasn't receiving signals from my eyes anymore. Using this concept, I attempted to manipulate my brain and eyes into reconnecting.

The blindness, however, was only a small part of what was wrong with my brain. I couldn't focus on anything, especially an obscure theory like rewiring the brain. It was so frustrating. It was as if a breaker had blown in my brain, and I was trying to turn the power on again. I went from a completely functioning, above average brain to not being able to find my butt with both hands. It just made sense to me that I could flip the switch back to the 'on' position. I had always been taught to take care of my own problems, not to sit around waiting for others to step up and do it for me. At that point no one else was offering assistance anyway. I never did figure out how to flip the 'switch'.

I continued to deal with these difficult experiences for many years.

Since the brain injury I also have horrible balance. This affects me most on stairs. I require a handrail to safely ascend or descend steps. Some of this, of course, is due to my limited vision but even with the aid of a rail my balance is so bad that I often experience instability on a flight of stairs.

To this day I have problems with my equilibrium. It comes and goes with no apparent trigger. When I am laying down and stand up too quickly I am dizzy and lightheaded. I cannot walk straight to save my life. Usually I list to the right. When this happens I have to be very careful not to fall down the stairs in my home, since they are just to the right of the hallway.

My coordination was greatly impacted by the brain injury. I am not able to learn specific dance moves. Over the years, I have had two different girlfriends attempt to teach me the Jitterbug, and my brain just can't connect to my feet. Before the brain injury, I participated in drill team at school. There were no problems with my coordination back then.

Something else I experienced that was due to my brain injury was problems with my body temperature. I always felt cold. I remember sitting outside in the sunshine on what should have been hot summer days but the slightest breeze felt cold to me and would give me chills. My dad would half-jokingly comment on me wearing my large, bulky letterman's jacket outside in an effort to stay warm on such days. To this day I still have difficulty with even slightly cool weather.

I also have some difficulty retaining information but have learned techniques to compensate for this. I have retained most of what I learned prior to the brain injury, but any new learning has been a challenge.

When it comes to hands on activities I learned before the tumor I enjoy complete recall. I also have very little trouble learning new hands on activities. Where I do have a snag is with new factual information; history and science in particular. Not surprisingly, perhaps, these are the only two subjects I had to make any effort to do well in at school prior to the tumor.

Several years ago I enrolled in the Montana School of Massage in Missoula. Being a massage therapist has been a long held dream of mine. I found, however, that I just could not retain the anatomy & physiology information required to complete the program. I also found kinesiology to be impossible due to my limited vision even though the school was willing to adapt the material for me. This was a huge disappointment in my life. It was one of the few things that I have attempted to do since the brain tumor that I just could not succeed at.

My tumor was discovered and removed when I was 12 years old, just as my body was preparing for me to enter puberty. As I entered this period of life, which is challenging under the best of circumstances, my sex drive was outrageous! I couldn't stop thinking about it. This continued for many years. Thinking back to the other kids around me, I am sure that my drive was abnormally enhanced in comparison.

I also had horrible social skills, a common symptom of brain injury. This caused me great difficulty with making or keeping friends, which in turn made my already lonely existence much more unbearable. My teenage years were very difficult for me.

Chapter Nine

I remember when some people came to our home from Visual Services in Havre. They had come to give me mobility and other training on how to function safely as a blind person. My mom chased them off our property. She was convinced she could take care of me the way I should be. There were no opportunities for me while I lived with her however. I needed to be in a larger community, where I had an opportunity to learn and become an independent person.

My mom would reason it out when she told me how she had chased these people away. She felt that only she could give me what I really needed but she was so very wrong. In our small town, I had no chance at all of any kind of fulfilling life. She was my mom and it was very hard to contemplate the need to flee when we had been so close before the tumor. Today it is surreal, looking back and realizing how desperate my situation was. All people, even disabled people, need to grow up and leave home. They can't be forced to remain childlike just to satisfy the needs of their parents.

Another part of living in Hingham that really made my life difficult was the layout of the town. The streets were gravel and covered in snow in the winter. I remember several occasions when I would be out walking, trying to find my way home, and I would get disoriented in the snow. I had grown up in Hingham and should have known my way around. When I regained a little vision and was trying to use it (since my mom wouldn't allow me to use my cane), I would often get lost in my home town. The problem I had was everything was white with snow. I couldn't see the difference between the road, ditches, yards or anything. I remember several occasions when I became lost for so long and grew so cold, I was afraid I would freeze before finally finding my way.

One day I was walking our family dog, Fred. We were walking through an abandoned lot where there had once been a bar. I fell into a deep hole and slid in all the way to my shoulders. This experience was very unsettling. I know, had I been provided with a white cane, my ability to mobilize safely would have been greatly enhanced. I would not have fallen in the hole.

I know I keep harping on the white cane. Many people view the white cane as something negative; a sign of disability. Rather, a white cane enables a blind person to safely navigate anywhere independently. I am a big proponent of using whatever tools one needs to enhance one's independence and safety. All of my friends and family can vouch for this.

When I was finally given the tools and training I had been denied by my mother, my life really turned around. I had found the independence I had always desired.

When a person has extremely low vision, and they are trying to walk without a white cane, it is heart-wrenching to watch. They shuffle their feet and stare at the ground. Some walk very slowly, and hold their hands out in front of themselves in an effort to prevent running into obstacles. They are afraid they will fall, stumble over an object, or run into something blocking their path. A white cane, with proper training, alleviates all of this. This tool also tells drivers that the person is low vision, thus making everyone safer. It provides safety and confidence to the blind when doing something as simple as walking.

Now that I have received a white cane and proper training, I am only dependent on said cane. With it I can go anywhere and do anything I want to. My dependence on my cane is so extreme that when I break it, as I do from time to time, I feel blind all over again. When using my cane I don't feel hindered by my blindness at all. Many people tell me they wouldn't believe I was blind when watching me travel with my cane. It is the increased confidence I experience when using my cane that they see.

This phenomenon of increased confidence bears an incredible impact on my safety when walking with my cane. When I travel independently away from home, whether on the greyhound bus or on an airplane, I take a second cane with me. I am so fiercely independent that I hate having to ask strangers for help.

On the topic of asking strangers, I have found that almost everyone I have come across has been willing to aid me if I ask. People sometimes fall all over themselves to help.

One day I was in downtown Missoula where I used to live. I was standing at an intersection, waiting for the proper time to cross. A total stranger came up behind me, looped his/her arm through mine, and proceeded to walk me across the intersection. They then released my arm. The person walked away without ever saying a word to me.

Unfortunately, I have talked to a lot of people who have tried to render aid to disabled people and have been met with hostility. I'm afraid that this causes some people to hesitate to help when it is actually needed. I find what works best for me is when someone believes I may need aid, they offer. Then I can gratefully accept, or thank them politely and refuse their help.

Just a few years ago I was at the bank, trying to make a payment on my credit card. The man in line behind me said something to me I didn't hear. I turned to face him and said "What?" He viciously cursed at me! I was shocked at his brutal treatment. I had done nothing to provoke such harsh words. I turned back to the teller who was helping me. She was a friend of mine and I had known her for several years. I was very upset by how I had just been treated. My eyes were brimming with tears. I was so embarrassed. I retrieved my receipt and left the bank.

As I left the bank and climbed into the car where my husband was waiting for me, I exclaimed, "I have never been treated so rudely!"

My husband could see that I was visibly upset and he demanded to know what had happened. I told him what the man had said to me. He went into the bank and demanded to know where the man was who had treated me so harshly. The teller's eyes grew large and she looked at the man. My husband turned to him and the man said in an effort to ward off my husband's wrath, "I'm disabled!" When my husband came back to the car and told me what had taken place in the bank I was so angry. Just because the man was "disabled" he felt he had the right to treat people with such disrespect! He felt bad when my husband told him I was blind but in my mind that was beside the point. Just because he was disabled didn't give him the right to treat *anyone* so offensively. He felt justified treating me that way when he didn't realize I was blind. I hope wherever he is today, the man no longer behaves uncivilized. There is no excuse for such behavior.

My husband was always fiercely protective of me. It made me feel really special.

I have found that I have a gift for asking people for help. I know what help I need and when I really need it. Sadly, many disabled people are too proud to ask for help and so they wind up looking foolish. People usually have more respect for a person who can admit when they may need a little help. We are all members of the human race and we must look after one another.

I have found that I am usually able to sense whether or not a person is "safe" to engage in conversation or interact with. This makes me feel a lot more comfortable when asking total strangers for assistance. I believe that this heightened sense of a person's character is just another benefit of my blindness.

In addition to dealing with the vicious attack from the jerk at the bank, I have also sustained violence from tree branches. As a white cane user, I find when walking, long tree branches that hang over sidewalks can be treacherous. It is dangerous to have tree branches hitting people in the face and eyes when they cannot see well.

Likewise, when walking on sidewalks, I find that snow-packed or icy walkways make it treacherous to safely travel in Missoula. Another issue with sidewalks: frequently I have had to dive out of the way to avoid being run down by skateboarders and bicyclists while walking on sidewalks downtown. I wish people would be more aware of the hazards pedestrians face, in particular blind pedestrians.

Some of my other observations regarding blindness have to do with eating out. For example, I sit at a table and it has a setting of not only plate and silverware; but also a saucer, soup bowl, coffee cup, water glass, and other beverage. Having all of these extra items in the way make it virtually impossible to enjoy a meal without spilling or breaking something. It would make it easier for me, as a blind person, if the wait staff would ask whether or not I'd like these additional items with my meal instead of just setting them before me.

There are many ways to make the dining experience for a blind person more functional. Some wait staff personnel give me a description of the location of the food on my plate using the face of the clock as a template. For example, they say things like: "Your meat is at 9:00, your vegetables are at 12:00, and your potatoes are at 3:00." This method works very well when helping a blind person understand the construction of the food on their plate. Not all wait staff is trained in this, however: just a friendly pointer. Then, there are buffets... I love the variety of options but it is literally impossible for me to use a buffet independently. I have found though, that if you ask the staff for assistance, they are usually willing and able to help you.

I have come face to face with common misconceptions regarding blindness. People have actually asked the question, "Why don't you just get glasses?" As if I wouldn't have thought of such a simple solution for this huge inconvenience on my own! When people ask me this question I almost laugh. It is quite ridiculous to think that I wouldn't already have glasses if they would help.

One of the huge challenges of being blind is my lack of fashion sense. I am in a constant state of "fashion nightmare." I, of course, am unable to see how other women are dressing and doing their hair and makeup. My attire typically consists of blue jeans, t-shirts, and tennis shoes. I do most of my clothes shopping at Wal-Mart. Hairstyle? Typically a pony-tail. Forget makeup! At this point in my life I am trying to improve my fashion sense. I have a few girlfriends now who I have been going shopping with to get a new wardrobe. I've been going to hair salons to get my hair highlighted. I even have a pair of snazzy shoes! When the weather is nice, I have a large number of beautiful summer dresses that I wear all the time. I am happiest when wearing my dresses.

When going shopping, I use the customer service staff at the stores to assist me. This works for grocery, clothes, or school supply shopping. When you have a list of specific items you are needing, they are extremely helpful in retrieving the items off the shelves for you. Christmas shopping is a whole different ball game! I find it impossible to browse the stores or the newspaper shopping ads looking for Christmas gifts for loved ones. This is one activity I have not found any viable solutions for. I typically end up buying exactly what people asked for. This is very frustrating. I would really like to be a creative gift giver.

There are so many ways my blindness has affected my life. One of the major psychological impacts it has had on me is my dreams. In the early years I would have dreams featuring my mother, my sisters, and other people that I knew well. During these dreams I would see the faces of these people. I could clearly see their faces because I had memories of what they looked like. Now, all these years later, those faces are fading. Today, I barely remember what my mother looks like. In truth, I have no idea what I look like; just the blurry image I see in the mirror. The friends and family members I know now, I have never "seen". In my current dreams, I no longer see faces. My dreams are made up of primarily emotions, sounds, and smells. For example, I'll dream of someone I care about and I'll know who they are because I sense them and hear their voice in my dream. I feel the emotions attached to that person. I can hear their voice. As far as nightmares go, in my nightmares it's not so much seeing bad things happening as feeling very frightened or alarmed. I know I've had a nightmare because of the distress I feel whenI wake up. Sometimes I know that the nightmare involved my children because I feel deep concern for their welfare.

People also talk about how they know what it is like to be blind when they close their eyes. This is nothing like being blind. When you close your eyes, you have the knowledge that you will see again once you open them. When you are blind and you open your eyes, you are still blind. Basically, when you are blind, you have to be constantly aware that you are not seeing your world correctly. You have to be acutely mindful of audio and tactile clues in your environment in order to keep yourself safe from danger. It is not a "lifestyle" I would recommend. It requires a great deal of focus.

In my case, medically speaking, my blindness is cortical. This means that my brain isn't receiving messages from my eyes. My brain doesn't translate what I am not seeing, much different than closing your eyes. I guess what I am saying is it is not exactly like seeing darkness, more like seeing nothing at all.

Actually, in my situation, I no longer see nothing at all. I can see light now and some very blurry shapes. I have been able to read for a number of years with my CCTV. This is a very expensive machine that blows up my print so I can see it better.

I also use my CCTV for balancing my checkbook and reading bills etc. I enjoy solving crossword puzzles with my CCTV. I find that working crosswords helps to keep my mental skills sharp. When I do crosswords I utilize my memory, concentration and attention.

My eyes have become quite tired after all these years though. I now attempt to get all my books on audio. I suffer a lot of headaches due to eye strain. I also have a lot of trouble with bright sunlight and the glare from the CCTV. My CCTV has a very bright light in it that enables me to see the print. It is frustrating that I require the light to see but it dries my eyes out and gives me headaches. I really miss taking a book with me wherever I go and just sitting down and reading it. When I go to a doctor's office I browse through the magazines in the waiting room, looking for large print headings I can read in order to help alleviate some of the boredom.

I have also discovered many tools for making computers and computer programs accessible to the blind. Freedom Scientific is a company that has created the JAWS program. JAWS is a program that talks to the computer user. It reads what is on the computer screen and anything the user enters on the keyboard. A blind person can utilize email and surf the web using JAWS. Some sites are easier to use than others, however. It is simply a matter of checking them out to see which ones work for you.

A blind person can also utilize Facebook using the JAWS program and going to m.facebook.com to set up a Facebook profile. Using this site, a blind person can enjoy and participate in Facebook using only the keyboard. When using m.facebook.com, a blind person participates in the same Facebook as the rest of the world. It is just a more accessible version of the popular site.

Chapter Ten

The day I graduated from Blue Sky was a day of mixed feelings. I was relieved to be done with it but I had no hope of any kind of independent or successful life. My mother had always chased the people off our property who came from Visual Services in Havre. They had come to teach me to live as a blind person. Joanne had also failed to get me treatment for my brain injury. I was forced to live with her for a year following high school. She did a good job keeping me dependent upon her.

In 1995, the year I graduated, I visited my father and stepmother in Minnesota for Christmas. A plan was hatched while I was there. I would move in with them. The promise was made that I would receive the training and tools I needed in order to live independently. My parents had good intentions. After I moved I discovered they didn't know where to find services. The mistake that all my parents made was they thought I needed to live with *them* in order to become independent. The opposite was actually true. Living with any of my parents forced me to remain dependent on them. Like I said, disabled people should not be forced to live with their parents.

In May of 1996, a year after graduating from high school, I moved in with my parents in Minnesota. When I lived in Minnesota with my dad and stepmother I was pretty much confined to my room. They had no idea what to do with me. My stepmother became so stressed out that she actually hired her friend to "babysit" me while she was at work. She

ordered this woman not to allow me to leave the house under any circumstances (keep in mind that I was 20 years old at this time.) My dad
and stepmom did allow me to get a phone line in my room, as if I knew
anyone I could call!

I wound up so lonely that I was calling a chat line I had heard about
from one of my half-brother's girlfriends.

Since the tumor I had been experiencing a very high sex drive. You
can probably guess what happened when they gave me a phone line of
my own and locked me in my room. That's right, I began having phone
sex. The chat line I had been calling was a local number so it didn't cost
me anything. There were plenty of men on the chat line who appreciated
getting it for free. I want to assure you that this was not my goal when
I asked for the phone line. That does seem to be the expected outcome,
however, given all the factors at hand.

I was very lonely and depressed. My relationship with my stepmother
had never been good, even before the tumor, and it was very strained
now. I continued living with my parents in Minnesota until early in 1997.

During this time my stepmom began taking me to see a doctor in
downtown Minneapolis. He also put me on drugs, specifically Prozac.
Again, it didn't benefit me at all. In fact my behavior became more
erratic. Once again, I want to point out that it was a bad situation, not a
chemical imbalance that was causing my behavior.

When we went to see the doctor we always went late at night. I
believe this was because my stepmom worked days.

My stepmom and this doctor cooked up a scheme to make me purchase a group home and then stick me in it. They tried to sell me on this
idea telling me that it would be a good investment and I would have
some amount of control there because it would be "mine."

I shudder today looking back at the situation. Talk about deceiving
and taking advantage of someone! I think my stepmom wanted to get
me out of her house. You can't blame her but where was I supposed to
go? I had no skills for living independently.

The circumstances in my stepmother's home became so hostile, I ran away one night while she was gone (if you can call it "running away.") I was over 18 after all and well within my rights to leave if I wanted to.

I called one of the people I had met through my brother. He came to the house, picked me up, and gave me a ride to a hotel. I stayed there for a couple of days.

My stepmother had herself added to my checking account as a signer and she held my checkbook so I couldn't spend my own money. I had, however, managed to get a debit card on my checking account and this was what I used to pay for my hotel room.

It was the closest motel to where my parents lived so they were pretty sure that's where I was staying. They couldn't be positive, however, because I had instructed the front desk to keep my presence from anyone who called asking after me.

My parents contacted the local police department. I spoke with an officer on the phone when I called my parent's house to speak to my brother. I agreed to tell the officer where I was but instructed him not to give the information to my parents. He agreed. I told him what room I was in at the hotel. The officer then came to see me.

When I opened the door to the officer, I stood in the doorway speaking with him. Several people were standing around gawking at what was happening. It was really surreal . I let him into my room. I sat on the bed and cried while I told him all about what it was like living with my stepmom. He probably thought I was a little nuts.

Later on as a stepmom myself of two teenagers I realized how normal my feelings were.

After a few days my dad came and picked me up from the hotel. He had made arrangements for me to go up north and stay with my grandma for a few days to give my stepmom and me a break. This sounded like a good idea but when I returned to my stepmom's house the situation remained the same. I was still confined to my bedroom. I could not leave the house without my stepmother's permission, and I had no friends.

That is when I planned a trip to Montana to visit my mom and stepdad.

I flew from Minneapolis to Great Falls with one of my stepmom's friends. This was the first time the woman had ever been to Montana and she really loved it. We rented a car in Great Falls and drove to Havre where we had reservations at a hotel. We stayed there while we were visiting my family in Hingham. Hingham is located about halfway between Havre and Chester on Highway 2.

I really enjoyed our trip. There was a casino in the hotel. I had never gambled before. My stepmom's friend helped me find a machine I could see a little bit. She taught me to play a couple of games on it. For the next few days, when I got bored, I would walk down to the casino and play a few bucks. It was a lot of fun walking around by myself and using the machine.

A couple of days after we had arrived there I won a Jackpot on the machine. This greatly excited me. I gambled quite a bit more money after that.

The woman I came with somehow met a couple of traveling salesmen while we were staying at the hotel. They were renting a house in Havre. Their roommate was a bouncer at a local bar.

The suggestion was made that we should all go to the bar and have some drinks. I was a few months shy of my 21st birthday at that time. When I informed them of this they told me not to worry; their roommate could get me in.

It is at this point I want to make sure you understand how impressionable I was. I had not been allowed to go out and have fun in high school. I had suffered an "arrested childhood." This suggestion greatly excited me so I went. I felt safe because I was with my stepmom's friend.

At the bar I drank a wine cooler. The bar was full of underage drinkers. I later found out that the bar had a reputation for serving minors. I danced with one of the salesmen and planted a lip lock on him. He and I had been intimate earlier (also a bad decision, but give me a break.)

My stepmother's friend and I went back to the hotel. I didn't realize at the time that I was enjoying my first and last fleeting moments of freedom. It was later that night when my reality once again spiraled out of control.

Part Three

Losing Everything I Had Left

Chapter Eleven

I was in my room at the hotel. It was evening. I am not sure where my traveling companion was at this precise moment. My mom and stepdad came into the room. This didn't surprise me. I figured my friend had allowed them into the room. I was there because I had been visiting them after all. Then my parents from Minnesota walked in. I immediately knew something was terribly wrong.

I began sobbing and said, "Oh my God! What's wrong? Who died?" (I figured if the situation was bad enough to get all my parents together, even the ones who lived so far away in Minnesota, it must be incredibly BAD).

My mother sat me down on the bed and explained that they were taking me to court to have her friend Pete Robertson appointed my guardian. This made no sense to me. Pete had been one of her lawyers who filed the original malpractice lawsuit. They had become *very* close over the years. I was confused and afraid. I did not understand what was happening. An "emergency" court hearing had been called before a judge in Havre whom I didn't know.

I was introduced to a man named Chevy and was told he would represent me in court. He was supposed to protect my rights as he was my "guardian ad litem." Then I was dragged into an emergency court hearing held late at night in Havre, Montana. At this time, I was a legal resident of the state of Minnesota. I was only in Montana for a visit.

I was so afraid and confused, I couldn't stop crying. It was utterly terrifying sitting there in court next to a total stranger, facing a judge whom I didn't know. The judge asked me if I understood what was happening. I knew I was in a courtroom; nothing else. I said I understood. The judge was presented with a recording of messages my mother had obtained off my voice mail in Minnesota. The judge was told that I had not only been telling the men I spoke to on the chat line how much money I had but that I had also been telling people I met in Havre. None of this was true but I was in no position to speak up for or defend myself. This was extremely embarrassing having the judge know I had engaged in phone sex. It is not something a person would like others to know. One of Pete's friends was allegedly in the bar that night. He had supposedly seen me kissing the man I was with and drinking a wine cooler. As if these actions were heinous crimes that should be held against me!

I was so embarrassed by all of this that I hung my head in shame. I couldn't show my face to the judge.

When you get right down to it, the only law I broke was drinking a wine cooler in the bar when I wasn't quite 21 years old. The judge believed everything he was told, however. As a result, he appointed Pete my "temporary" guardian.

This appointment was supposed to last for only six months. It began in February of 1997. Pete made sure to get me back into the judge's courtroom in August of that year before his temporary appointment lapsed. He then had himself appointed my full permanent guardian. I had no representation in court that day. I was still in Bridges, and working on the process of recovering. Pete took full advantage of my vulnerability.

As a result of this court action my private property was seized and I was stripped of my civil rights. It may be hard for you to understand what this means but I will make it clear in the coming pages.

Part Four

The Approaching Dawn

Chapter Twelve

*O*n February of 1997, no sooner had he been appointed my "temporary" guardian, Pete promptly brought me to Missoula, Montana to enter the Community Bridges Program.

Bridges is a traumatic brain injury rehabilitation program that is affiliated with Community Medical Center. This program, as it turned out, was exactly what I needed. Bridges was the treatment for my brain injury that my mom had denied me for years. I remember around the time the lawsuit was settled over-hearing my mom speak about the program. She had found out about it from her attorneys. Looking back, I can only imagine how events in my life would have turned out differently had she allowed me to attend the Community Bridges Program all those years ago.

This extraordinary and amazing program was *the* significant turning point in my recovery.

The first day I came to Bridges, I was frightened and overwhelmed. I was still reeling from the horrific experiences I had in court. Everything I owned was still in Minnesota, but I was not allowed to return to my home. We met with a group of strangers at Community Hospital. Several of the people in the meeting were doctors and therapists. They were all wearing white lab coats. The rooms in the hospital all looked white to me with my limited vision. I truly believed Pete was sticking me in an institution. Why wouldn't I suspect Pete was capable of this? His friend, my mother, had threatened to do the same for years whenever I would raise any protest to her use of my funds.

After the meeting at the hospital we all went to look at the residential side of the program. Back then the residential dorms were located at an apartment complex on Cooper Street.

I remember how in awe I was when I saw where I would be living. I was to have an apartment of my very own! Apparently the apartments were sub-standard, judging from what my mothers were saying while we had our tour. but I was thrilled! It was my first independent living situation. I was to cook and clean for myself.

This was more freedom than I had ever been allowed to experience.

My four parents were along for the tour. My two moms promptly decided that this wouldn't do, I could not be put in an apartment of my own without close supervision.

I, on the other hand, was elated. I informed them that there was nothing they could do about it now, they had Pete appointed my guardian and *he* wanted me there.

The staff at the Bridges program warned me that if I ran away, they would place me in the Providence Center, which is a lock-down facility. Everyone was so ignorant about why I said and did the things I said and did. I had run away from a horrible situation when I was in Minnesota at my step-mother's house. Bridges was offering me what I had always longed for. Why would I run away from the opportunity to learn and prove myself capable at last? It's really sad to think about today; the way they had me constantly trying to live up to their expectations for my life. I still find myself trying to please others and not myself. I am my own worst critic though so I perform the best when trying to live up to my own expectations.

After the orientation to the program, my four parents went back to their respective homes and Pete went back to Havre where he lived. Havre is 281 miles northeast of Missoula. It didn't occur to me back then that it wasn't right Pete was so far away from me while maintaining complete control over my life and happiness. I would come to the realization years later how a guardian's power can be abused.

Chapter Thirteen

$\mathcal{I}$ settled into my apartment that first night and met several of the staff members. I still remember how exciting it was sleeping in my own apartment. The staff members were very nice. The clinicians worked primarily at the hospital and the LSTs (Life Skills Trainers) usually worked at the apartments.

In the mornings I would awaken independently with the aid of an alarm clock. I would shower and get ready for the day. The LSTs would come to my apartment to check in on me. I was expected to have a game plan for the day figured out. During the week we (the clients) would ride in the van to the hospital where we would take part in groups designed to aid our brains in beginning to function efficiently again. We also had one on one counseling sessions with a doctor at the hospital about once a week.

I remember several of the groups. REB was the group I enjoyed the most. It was taught by one of my favorite staff members. She was awesome. She also led Women's Group which was a support group for women with TBI (Traumatic Brain Injury). There was Men's Group for the guys also.

REB stood for Rational Emotive Behavior. In this group we were first taught how to examine our thoughts to determine if they were logical. Next we would look at how these thoughts affected our emotions. Then we would look at how our emotions would influence our behavior. In this group we were also taught how to take ownership of our emotions, how to "decide" to be in control of how we felt when a person did or said something to us. For example, if someone said or did something to us that was, for lack of a better word, "unfair", we could now prevent them from "making" us feel a certain way. We were in control of how we would react. This may sound rather elementary to someone who hasn't sustained a brain injury but when you are living with a TBI this process gets really muddled up. This was one of my biggest problems. What I learned in REB empowered me.

In Bridges we also learned about various types of brain injuries. There are closed-brain injury, and open-brain injury. An open-brain injury is where the skull is fractured or open in some way. A closed-brain injury occurs when the brain is damaged but the skull remains intact. My brain injury was both an open-brain/closed-brain injury. The pressure of the tumor and everything that happened to my brain before the surgery was the closed-brain injury. The act of drilling into my skull and cutting into my brain to remove the tumor was the open-brain part of my injury. Each injury was very traumatic in its own way.

People may not think about this, but a concussion is also a brain injury and thus should be treated as such. Many people go about their daily lives after a concussion not realizing there may be residual damage to their brain. Another example of common brain injury is a stroke.

Some brain damage symptoms are easy to recognize, while other symptoms are less obvious to the world.

Another part of the program that I have found particularly helpful was how we were taught to communicate. A person can be passive, aggressive, assertive or a combination of passive and aggressive.

When I came to Bridges I was a passive communicator but I learned to be assertive. I am much happier as an assertive person.

I use the skills I learned in REB all the time in my marriage and in raising my sons. I teach my children how to use these skills when they have disagreements between themselves and when they come home from school angry with their friends or teachers. I think that if people all learned how to use REB before they got married there would be far less divorces.

As I said, Bridges was exactly what I needed to recover. It is a good program for people in that situation but there is something else I need to point out.

A person will not succeed at Bridges if the time is not right. For example, I met a man who was accepted into the program. He was confined to a wheelchair and had a severe head injury. I befriended him. He did not successfully complete the program however. He went into a group home when he left. In my opinion, they should have waited until he was done with the grieving process and was ready to apply himself to getting better before they accepted him. He may have been able to live independently after the program had he been in a position to make the effort to get better. Instead he was still grappling with his handicap. I remember he would spend a lot of his time at the day program crying over his situation.

One day it happened. The day when the "click" occurred for me was profound. I was sitting in the day program, participating in a group when I suddenly realized I was able to think clearly once again. I was able to focus on what was being said and process the information. It was exhilarating! Up until this point, my brain just didn't function properly. The effects of my brain injury made me feel as if I was drunk all of the time. When the "click" occurred, it was as if the heavy veil that encompassed my mind was lifted. I was able to correctly perceive my world once more. No one told me I could ever feel like this again. I look at this as a significant event in my recovery.

In the residential side of the program, LSTs would work with us on tasks of daily living, i.e. making a grocery list or to-do list, organizing our living environment, and making our daily/weekly schedules. The staff members also had us setting goals and tracking our progress toward achieving them.

In all things the entire staff was constantly practicing positive feedback with the clients.

The program was designed to create a world in which we always had opportunities not only to learn but to practice the skills we were learning. It was complete immersion in the program and I thrived on it all.

The staff at Bridges also connected me with the local Visual Services office through the county government. Through Visual Services I received mobility training. I was given lessons on how to cook and do other tasks involved in daily living as a blind person. This essential training was one of the things my mother had denied me. This was also a significant step in gaining my independence.

I made a lot of good friends at Bridges. The behaviorist with the program was one of my favorites. He treated me like an equal and I remember times when he would bounce hypothetical situations off me to see what I thought he should do. He would then listen attentively to my ideas and the reasoning behind them. This caused me to feel like my opinion mattered.

One of the LSTs, who was eventually promoted to Transitional Living Coordinator, was also a good person. He always joked around with us clients when he was an LST and also when he became the TLC.

I was very driven to succeed in Bridges. A big reason for this was the LSTs. They were all, more or less, in their twenties and I quickly became friendly with several of them. I felt like I had friends for the first time in a very long time. The LSTs were young, smart, healthy people; everything I wanted to be. They practiced positive feedback with the clients and I responded to this with a new found drive to make my life good again.

I had suffered such negativity from my parents for years. I just couldn't do anything right. Under the positive reinforcement at the Bridges program, I flourished.

The LSTs and I became such close friends that they often shared the inner circle gossip with me. For example, I knew who was sleeping with whom. The girl who told me this was the girl who was doing the sleeping with one of the male staff members. I didn't hear it second hand so I took it seriously. The male staff member was also a friend. When I hinted to him that I knew what he had been doing, he was very nervous. I also knew which staff member was sleeping with a former client.

Along with social benefits, I was also experiencing physical fulfilment. When I came to Bridges I participated in Body Shop. During Body Shop they would usually take us to the YMCA to work out. I wasn't in bad shape when I came to Bridges but I became physically fit working out regularly. I quickly began spending much of my free time at the Y.

Looking back I think I was addicted to the endorphins my body was manufacturing when I worked out. A person can certainly have worse addictions.

I remember my mom's reaction when she came to visit me the first time. Family and friends couldn't visit for a while after a person entered the program. I was tanned and had great muscle tone on my arms and legs. She was in awe of me. I think at that point she probably realized that Bridges was a good place for me.

The summer I was in Bridges there were cut backs in Medicaid. Several of the clients had to leave and the employment of many staff members was terminated. This was very difficult for me. I had grown fond of so many of them. I have always felt that Bridges is a very unique and essential program. It changes lives and our society for the better. I remember being so lonely for a time that summer. At one point I was the only client in the program.

Chapter Fourteen

*A*nd then there was Bill. I met Bill in Bridges. He was one of several clients I became friends with in the program. I am not sure how he sustained his brain injury or when he entered the program. He had gone to culinary school at some point prior to me knowing him. On Thursdays we had "Community Dinners" prepared by the clients. He and I were sometimes assigned the task of organizing and cooking the meal. We all took turns. This was just one of the events in which Bill and I worked closely.

I remember one night there was a knock on my apartment door. I said "Who is it?" A voice on the other side of the door identified himself as Bill. When I opened the door he told me about a problem he was having with his laundry. For some unknown reason he was developing large bleach spots on his jeans. He was wondering if I was having the same problem. As it turned out, he was using the wrong soap for his laundry. He was using the dish washer detergent instead of the laundry soap! Both were available in unmarked tubs in the LST office. This interaction is one of my favorite memories involving Bill. He was so sheepish when he came to my apartment that night to talk to me.

There was something about Bill. I began developing feelings for him. He made it clear to me that he had similar feelings. I smile today, looking back at some of the spontaneous, romantic things he would say and do when he was around me. My favorite memory is of the time he popped up out of nowhere and swept me into his arms; passionately kissing me. He told me in that moment he would come back for me and take me to Mexico with him someday. He was older than me but that never mattered to either of us.

We wound up engaging in a physical relationship while I was still in the program. I was head over heels in love with him. You may be thinking I was merely experiencing first love; that Bill was my first lover and therefore I was too inexperienced to recognize true love. This was not the case. Bill was far from the first man I had entered into a physical relationship with.

Ultimately, I wound up emotionally distraught. The behavior that Bill and I were engaging in was against the rules of the program. I felt great anguish that Bill and I had to sneak around and did not have the freedom to be open about our relationship. I felt certain the staff would force us to never see each other again if anyone found out. I am sure the staff members with the program were concerned about what was happening to me. My demeanor and my overall outlook on life changed drastically. They did not know what was going on between Bill and me.

Bill could also see that I was having difficulties. He told one of the doctors with the program what we had been doing. I had always been made to feel by my parents that I wasn't good enough for a man to want and should never have sex. I was very troubled when Bill did this but looking back I can see it was what needed to be done to help me at the time. He only did it because he cared. I truly loved Bill and I believe he also loved me.

When he came clean to the powers that be about what we had been doing, someone decided that Bill and I shouldn't have the right to ever pursue a relationship with each other. They threatened to press charges against him for statutory rape if he didn't leave me alone. They got away with this because as far as the state was concerned, I was equal to a minor child in need of protection. Bill couldn't stay away though. I remember him stopping by the day program to check on me a couple of times after that.

As a result of my relationship with Bill, before I transitioned out of the program, a stipulation was made. I was taken against my will by some of the staff members to a women's clinic in Missoula. I was forced to undergo a medical procedure to implant a device in my body that prevented pregnancy. I was so traumatized at how I was treated. Pete never discussed this with me at all; he just had them do it to me. He was such a coward. He never discussed anything with me regarding my situation. I felt like a piece of meat during his guardianship. He acted like I didn't have any feelings or even the ability to form an opinion about anything.

As a result of this demoralizing and invasive procedure, I wound up feeling extremely violated. I never could set foot in that women's clinic again.

Pro-Choice advocates are always ranting about women's rights, but when this horrific experience was forced upon me, they were nowhere to be found. They were missing in action when I needed them most.

After I had undergone the medical procedure, I was allowed to transition out of the residential program. I was now able to find my own residence in Missoula. Even though I was discharged from the program, I still had round the clock babysitters hired by Pete. He was still in Havre and so out of touch with me, he needed to make sure I was safe.

One night, one of the babysitters took me to see Bill and we were able to spend a complete night together; our first and last. The next day Bill moved away.

It was 1999 when I ran into Bill on the streets in Missoula. We only exchanged a few words and embraced once but it was so good seeing him again. I have no idea where he is now.

Dr. Harris Johnson was the doctor whom Bill told of our relationship. While counseling me about my relationship with Bill, Dr. Johnson asked me if I knew what Bill looked like. Of course I didn't. It didn't matter to me what Bill looked like. Dr. Johnson proceeded to inform me that Bill was Mexican, as if this should impact my feelings for him. This really made me angry. What did race have to do with it? Race should never matter in a relationship. We are all God's children. Dr. Johnson's use of his own personal view during his treatment of me struck me as very unprofessional and extremely unethical.

Chapter Fifteen

When I transitioned out of Bridges, Pete initially hired LSTs from the program to baby sit me around the clock. While on duty, these LSTs would document my behavior. They would write down everything I chose to do or not to do. For example, if I chose to postpone unloading my dishwasher that day, they would write it down. If I chose to leave a basket of clean laundry on the couch instead of folding it right away, they would document that as well. Every choice I made was judged and written down. They wanted to see if I was making "good decisions". The anxiety created by this constant judging of every choice I made became incredibly stressful.

It was during this time that I was introduced to marijuana. There were a lot of new "friends" in my life at that point. Man those were crazy days!

When I smoked marijuana I had some very interesting experiences. My eyes would dilate like other people's eyes. This made my limited field of vision so much larger and made it easier for me to see. Some people have hallucinations when they smoke marijuana. When I would take a hit, I knew the instant the drug would reach my brain because what I was looking at in that precise moment would instantly come into sharper focus, very much like using a microscope. Everything I saw when I was stoned appeared in bright colors, thus making my environment clearer. The bad part of smoking the drug was that I had a lot of difficulty concentrating on what was going on around me.

I remember when my friends and I would go to my favorite Mexican restaurant here for dinner after we had been smoking. My friends would be tripping out. They were convinced that the staff at the restaurant (most of whom know me personally) knew that we were stoned. The staff was coming out of the kitchen and gawking at us, according to my friends. I struggled to figure out how likely it was that my acquaintances at the restaurant were aware of our mutual state of mind. I couldn't determine if this was likely because I couldn't concentrate. I experienced these difficulties concentrating all the time when I was stoned so I decided I couldn't do it. It was more important to me that I could take care of myself than to experience the benefits from the drug.

I am a supporter of legalizing marijuana. My hope is that the FDA may be able to study the drug and remove the parts of the drug that hamper cognitive function while leaving the beneficial effects. So many medical advances are being made through science at the cellular level; perhaps they can also break down the marijuana plant and manipulate it.

After this period of time I went home to where my parents and my sister Lynn lived. I wanted to be there when my sister had her first child. When I came back to Missoula Pete hired a home health care agency to babysit me around the clock.

While with this agency, I wound up smoking marijuana with four members of their staff who were being paid to watch me. For just over two months I was stoned almost every waking hour. I realized that I was unable to stop smoking because so many of the people Pete had hired were bringing it to work with them, intending to smoke with me. When I first decided to stop I couldn't. It was all around me every day. These four staff members had volunteered to take all the extra shifts they could get with me because of the accessibility to drugs when they worked with me. When I tried to "change my playpens and playmates" I couldn't get away from them.

I called Pete and confessed to what had been going on. He promptly had his sister who lived in Missoula come over to my house and take me back to Bridges where I would be safe until he could decide what to do with me.

Pete was so lucky. He had lived here previously and had friends and family here. This gave him the ability to accomplish many things even though he was so far away. I became fed up with hearing from him "I know someone there who can..." He was the one collecting a paycheck from my account but he was always delegating things to other people because he couldn't be here himself. I wound up paying not only Pete, but so many of his friends and family to achieve his agenda.

Chapter Sixteen

The time I spent in Bridges when I reentered the program was basically just a wash. I had already completed the program. Pete just stuck me there in order to keep me safe.

While Pete was trying to decide what to do with me, the suggestion was made that I should buy a house for my stepdad and mom so they could move to Missoula. I would live in a trailer behind the house where I would have some level of privacy. At first this sounded reasonable to me. I quickly realized, however, what it would ultimately mean.

I would once again be completely at the mercy of my mother. She had never supported my independence before, and I was sure she would be the same. Her disdain for my independence was so bad that when I was at her house on my 21st birthday she told me "If you are "lucky", I will "let" you go uptown and buy a drink today since it's your birthday." This remark was a perfect example of how Joanne had always treated me. I was not allowed to have any rights or privileges unless she permitted it. I didn't get that drink. I didn't want it, I wasn't a drinker. Maybe I should have taken her up on her kind offer if only to exercise my right since she was offering to give it to me.

I went to Dr. Johnson when I realized that the most recent plan would not work. He was at the time in support of the idea, since it was the only one being offered. I expressed my concerns to him and he immediately saw my issue with the plan. He informed Pete that it was not a good idea so the plan was taken off the table.

I remember being shocked the way Dr. Johnson took my concerns so seriously. I expected him to blow me off, as usual. I had always been treated that way by all the members of the "team." It was really stupid, they were always making decisions for me and about me but not allowing me to have any input.

Eventually, Dr. Johnson brought Marjory Hartford on board to be my case manager. He was familiar with her work through former contact.

The first time I met Marjory was when she came to Bridges to see me. I was taken into a private room to meet with her. After she talked to me a little bit she laid hands on me and prayed for me. This was far out! No one had ever done this to me before.

She seemed nice enough so I gave my consent to her becoming my case manager, although I doubt it would have mattered if I had protested.

When Marjory was hired it made things more convenient for Pete. He now had someone on the ground here that he could depend on to take care of things for him. For me, it made things much more difficult. I could only communicate with Pete through Marjory after this.

Pete still didn't want me alone so his sister found a woman named Betty to live with me.

Betty and I moved into a house in the lower Rattlesnake, a very beautiful part of town. She had a bedroom in the finished basement and I slept upstairs. Betty had a life of her own though so she couldn't be expected to babysit me all the time. Marjory hired some of her friends and some of Betty's friends to pick up the slack. These were, for the most part, nice people and none of them were smoking marijuana in my house. I had no privacy though. Betty felt that it was alright for her to enter my bedroom without my consent. She only went in to gather my laundry and go wash it. I was perfectly capable of doing my own laundry though and I felt violated by her invasion of my privacy. When I discussed this with her however, she understood my feelings on the matter. She agreed to no longer enter my bedroom without my permission.

I think Betty thought that she was being hired to take care of me. For all I know, this could be what Pete told her. I was not privy to the arrangements he had made with her. Pete never did get a grip on what was going on with me. He just collected a paycheck from my account and tried to keep things functioning here so he could do his own thing in Havre.

Over time Marjory began cutting back on the hours the babysitters were at my house. I remember Pete was very stressed out by this. Marjory told me he was concerned. She continued to cut back hours though.

Eventually they were all gone and I just had to call Marjory to check in and let her know when I left my house and call her again to let her know when I returned. This was very liberating for me; imagine this after being a virtual prisoner all my life? I think though that all the phone calls became quite burdensome on Marjory. After a while I had to leave her messages because she wasn't available. I was just playing the game and doing what I had been told to do. Eventually she told me I didn't need to call her and check in anymore.

During this time, while Marjory was cutting hours, Betty wound up moving out of my house. I no longer had anyone at night. I am not sure what happened between Marjory and Betty but I remember Betty felt slighted by Marjory's actions. She seemed to want me to take sides between the two of them but I felt caught in the middle. I liked Betty. We had different beliefs and I know this was one thing that caused a problem between her and Marjory but I didn't care what Betty's beliefs were. She was good to me.

In July of 1999 Marjory forced me to sign up for a college course. Public speaking was selected.

During this month a whole semester of schooling was crammed into four weeks. I was so overwhelmed. I did not receive any assistance from the disabled student's services on campus. Marjory did not know what she was doing. I had a terrible experience that month. The final outcome was that I wound up hating school and feeling like a complete failure.

Two of the babysitters could see how much trouble I was having. They spent so many hours with me, trying to study. All three of us were incredibly overwhelmed. Of course Marjory wasn't around much to hear our complaints.

There was a man I met through Marjory. I would see him at her house. One evening he came to my house uninvited. I thought he was safe so I let him in when he knocked on my door. He entered into my kitchen and began aggressively shoving me backward. His behavior terrified me. I was all alone and he was much stronger than me. He was talking very strange, like he had been using a substance. Judging from what he was saying, he seemed to be upset with me for some reason, although I had no idea why.

I somehow managed to talk him into leaving my home. I still don't know how. He was definitely in control of the situation, I wasn't. I never found out what his agenda was when he showed up that night.

When he left I called Marjory and told her what had happened. I don't know what she did about it but he never acted inappropriately toward me again. It was, however, very uncomfortable for me seeing him at her house after that. He gave me the creeps. He had acted like a loose cannon, and I was never sure after that what he might do to me.

Another peculiar part of the situation with Marjory was that her step-daughter was an employee of the home health care agency that was hired to babysit me. Her step-daughter was one of the employees who was supplying me with marijuana and smoking with me. What a small community Missoula was!!

Marjory was always telling me stories that gave me the impression she was quite an authority on all things related to the Bible. She told me about doing "spiritual warfare" for God against demons and witches. She told me about her ex-husband. She said he was her "Saul" and that God was going to bring him back to her, even though he had remarried.

She was also convinced that one of her daughters was called to be a mighty warrior for God.

She invited me to her house for weekly church meetings. At these meetings we would walk the streets of her neighborhood, "praying for the land." We were "breaking spiritual curses off the land." She and her friends were "taking the land back from the enemy."

On December 31st, 1999 I was with Marjory and her friends. It had been prearranged that we would get together and pray/walk her neighborhood on that significant night.

There had been a huge build up to this date in the media. It was the Y2K bug. Everything was supposed to crash at midnight. I figured that if everything did crash I would be better off with people than at home alone.

I have to admit that I didn't see any harm in what Marjory and her friends were doing. They weren't hurting anyone or damaging property, but I think it was rather unprofessional of her to introduce me to these unorthodox beliefs.

At the time I was a sponge, soaking up whatever I could of the world around me. Marjory took full advantage of my vulnerability. She discussed with me that she believed that God had given me my money so I could use it for His will and she was the one who could tell me what His will was.

This greatly concerned me. I knew it wasn't a good idea to seek or receive any financial advice from her.

One time I asked Marjory how much I was paying her. I figured I should be entitled to this information since it was my funds that were paying her salary. She absolutely refused to tell me what her hourly rate was or to let me see her billing statements. I felt very suspicious about her keeping this information from me.

One of Marjory's friends who was working in my house back then was seeing demons. When I talked to Marjory about this, she told me that the woman was also a "spiritual warrior."

This woman often drove me around town. She spent so much time praying over other drivers that I was seriously concerned for my safety. It just didn't seem like she was paying enough attention to her own driving.

Although Marjory did some pretty ridiculous things to me, she was the first person to give me an opportunity to prove that I could take care of myself and I will always be grateful to her for this. I shudder to imagine where I would be today if Pete was still in control of my life.

Chapter Seventeen

*B*efore Marjory got rid of all the babysitters, they were the only people I ever hung out with. One of them, who was a friend of Marjory's, invited me to church.

At the church there was a revival going on. I was open to whatever God wanted to do in my life and I wound up baptized in the Holy Spirit. During this experience I felt overcome with the presence and the knowledge of the Lord in my spirit. I felt such a close union with the Lord that I knew he would hear my prayers when I prayed. I have always believed that God created someone for everyone so I began praying for my husband.

Since I had grown up, whenever I would meet someone new, I would wonder, "Could he be the one God created for me?" When I began praying for a husband, I stopped looking for him so it was very surprising how God brought us together.

I remember it vividly; I was sitting in church on a Wednesday night in January of 1999 when a woman sitting in front of me turned around and inquired, "Haven't I seen you on the bus?" I told her she probably had because I took the bus as well. I proceeded to give her a long list of my favorite places to go on the bus, one of which was my volunteer job at the food bank.

The guy sitting next to her said, "Wow, you work at the food bank? I wish I could do that."

He was her son, Randi. It turned out that Randi had been blinded thirteen months before this meeting and he had been a diligent construction worker prior to becoming disabled. His wife had walked out on him when he had gone blind. His mom had moved over from Washington to help him with his two small children after his wife had left. He was spending his entire time sitting at home playing video games.

I told him that if he would meet me at the courthouse on Friday I would take him to the food bank with me and introduce him to my boss, the volunteer coordinator.

Ultimately, we got to know each other over several months while we worked together at the food bank and spent many additional hours together each week hanging out around town. We began to develop feelings for each other. We professed our love for each other and we began "dating."

While we were getting to know each other, Randi was prayed for by the pastor one night in church. The next morning he awoke and read to his mom out of the Bible.

Over the following months his vision gradually improved until the doctor proclaimed he had 20/20 vision.

Randi and I had known each other for almost two years when I went to Minnesota for ten days to visit my family. We talked on the phone so much while I was gone. We missed each other terribly. I was staying with my grandma while I was in Minnesota. While I was there, I used my phone card so I wouldn't run up her bill. Boy, my phone bill was huge when I got it.

When I returned home Randi came to my house and asked me to marry him. I said I would. It seemed like the right thing to do, get married, so we could be together forever.

Randi's proposal caused me some anxiety though. I knew that because of my financial situation I would have to require him to sign a prenuptial agreement. This is a difficult topic to discuss with someone you plan to marry and spend the rest of your life with. If you can't trust them to not take advantage of you, how can you expect them to trust *you?*

So I sat him down one day and told him about my money. I was shocked to find out that he already knew. My mother, Joanne, had told him the first time she had met him when I had taken him home to meet my family.

Gee, talk about a hypocrite! If he had any ill intent toward me, she had set me up for him to take full advantage of me. It didn't surprise me though, she was always telling people about the money. She liked people knowing that she had access to a lot of it. The money caused a lot of problems for Randi and me when we were getting to know each other.

During our engagement we suffered a lot of judgment from our friends and family at church. They judged us because Randi had been married before and had gone through a divorce, forget the fact that many of them were divorced and remarried themselves. They also thought Randi was just marrying me for my money. We also had to jump through hoops to keep Pete happy. Pete and everyone else couldn't fathom that someone would want to marry me for just who I was. They were so sure that Randi had ulterior motives despite all the evidence to the contrary.

We just wanted to get married. What was with all the shenanigans? To this day, I am surprised Randi didn't turn tail and run screaming when he found out about the insanity of these people.

I remember during that time I was so frustrated. Pete and everyone else acted like I should have checked the balance of Randi's bank account before I got to know him. They were all so focused on the damn money. Is this normal behavior? I think not.

Randi and I began premarital counseling with our pastor, who is a licensed premarital counselor with the state of Montana. Pete insisted that we also receive premarital counseling from Dr. Harris Johnson, a neuropsychologist with the Bridges Program.

I only agreed to this because Pete had laid down the law. I had no choice. Pete had forced me to see Dr. Johnson for years. I had begged Pete to allow me to stop seeing Dr. Johnson because I always felt worse when I would leave his office than before I would go in. I would learn years later why this was.

This counseling was a really dumb and costly experiment. It was like going to a plumber to get dental work done, just another one of Pete's idiotic ideas.

Pete refused to permit me to get married until Dr. Johnson said it was okay.

Dr. Johnson finally gave his permission for us to get married after I told him why I thought we could make it work. I pointed out all the obstacles Randi and I had overcome alone as well as those we had conquered together. I also pointed out that we couldn't possibly wind up facing anything worse after we were married.

Dr. Johnson told Pete we could get married after this appointment. How nice, they decided to "let" a twenty-four year old woman get married! This greatly angered me. Why did I need Dr. Johnson's permission to get married? I'll tell you why: Pete was so far away and out of touch with what was going on with me he just couldn't make the judgment call himself.

At this point I must say that the worst obstacles we have had to overcome in our marriage were the direct result of the guardianship. It is not natural for a guardianship to be set between a man and his wife. It was like a large, invisible monster right there, driving a wedge between my husband and me.

We got married on June 16th 2001. We had been wed in a private ceremony prior to this however so we would not be living in sin when we moved in together. After our private ceremony I went to a doctor and had the device removed from my body which Pete and his cronies had forced me to get long ago. On our wedding day, I was pregnant.

When we finally had our wedding ceremony, Randi and I both felt that a lot of people who were present at our wedding were counting on us not lasting more than a few months. Boy, they misjudged us if that was what they were thinking. Today, we have been married for sixteen years.

I still remember how I felt three months later on September 11th, 2001 when our country was attacked. I was newly married, and was very apprehensive about what was going to happen to our country. My heart was overcome with dread for my unborn baby. What kind of world would my child grow up in?

Chapter Eighteen

After I got married Marjory did some really nutty things. On one occasion she accompanied my mobility instructor and me on a lesson. During the lesson, he told her about how the yellow painted curbs helped someone with my limited vision see the curb to prevent tripping on it. This also helps a person with limited vision to identify the corner of the sidewalk. It is very helpful when mobilizing around downtown with a white cane and limited vision.

She took this piece of information and decided that I should paint the floor of my laundry room florescent orange to make it easier for me to see laundry that I might inadvertently drop on the floor when I was washing clothes. She told my husband shortly after we got married that he would have to paint the floor.

When my husband asked me if it was really necessary to do this, I couldn't stop laughing at Marjory's ignorance.

I assured my husband that it was not. If I should have any need for contrast on my laundry room floor, a colored rug would be sufficient. It didn't occur to Marjory that this contrast only worked when there was sufficient difference between the color of the surface and the color of the contrast. This was a great solution for curbs downtown but it would offer very little benefit on my laundry room floor.

Marjory was really dangerous with her foolish ideas. She would take a small amount of information and act on it as if she had sufficient training in a certain area. Of course, she didn't. During the time she was my case manager, I wound up in some very uncomfortable predicaments due to her lack of experience. Pete gave Marjory complete control over everything going on in my life and I sometimes felt like I wound up in dangerous situations because of it.

Another one of Marjory's crazy ideas was about food. She decided that I should put together thirty casseroles at the beginning of each month. I should then freeze all thirty casseroles. Then, throughout the month I could simply remove one casserole from the freezer each night and bake it for my family.

It didn't occur to her that I couldn't afford to buy all the food required for such an undertaking or that I didn't have extra room in my freezer for thirty casseroles. Strangely, my house was not equipped with a commercial sized kitchen for this project either. When I called Pete to ask for extra money to facilitate Marjory's idea he refused to give me the money so I had to tell her no.

After I got married Marjory had some of her friends working in my new house again. A very bad situation developed with one of them.

My son began demonstrating behavior that made me think someone was abusing him. The only new person in his life at the time was Marjory's friend. When I told Marjory of my concerns for my child's safety, she had a cow. This was her friend we were talking about after all. I guess it was unreasonable for me to expect her to decide between the two of us. She refused to entertain my concerns. This really upset me. Why did I have to let this woman in my house; around my child? Why was Pete allowing this to go on?

I couldn't call Pete about it myself because if I should dare to call him, he always flew into a rage. He said he wanted Marjory to take care of things here; he was too busy to be bothered with my needs. This was the man I was being forced to pay thousands of dollars to in order to "protect" me and mine. He didn't care about me though. He only wanted to protect the money. I always felt like I was just in his way.

During the time this was going on with Marjory's friend, my husband came to me and told me he was very uncomfortable. The husband of Marjory's friend had been approaching him on the sly, attempting to convince him to talk to me about investing with his company.

I found this appalling. How had Marjory found out about my financial situation? Clearly she had told her friend about it.

It is a miracle that my family and I were not harmed any worse when Marjory was in charge. She completely trusted people she met if they were church going folks. There was more than one shady character I ran into that I met through Marjory. Most of them I only met because she hired them to work in my house around my family. Any of these friends of Marjory's could have done any number of horrible things to us and I was forced to allow them here. I was so frustrated with the situation we were put in due to Pete's lack of concern for me.

When Marjory's friends were working in my house some of our possessions were disappearing. It was virtually impossible to keep people from stealing from us. Randi was at work all day and I was low vision so I couldn't see what people were doing when they were in my home. With all the other stuff that was going on though, this was the least of my concerns at the time. I had a child to protect.

I think the thing Marjory did to me that upset me the most was when she tried to force me to do what was against my morals.

After my son was born she started riding me about getting out of the house. She wanted me to find a day care to stick my son in and go get a job. I had never worked before I got married but now all of a sudden she wanted me to do this. I think she wanted to impress Pete with the fact that she could also employ me.

This really upset me. I wanted to raise my son, not let strangers do it. I have always felt strongly that children are better off being raised by their parents than by strangers.

Marjory was always trying to force her religious and feminist beliefs on me. These two schools of thought are so opposite each other though, I think this was why her ideas never worked. I remember that her solution when I would have disagreements with my stepchildren or my husband was always to kick them out of my house. She was all about trying to destroy my family and marriage, not to help us make it work.

This backfired on her though. Because of what we had to go through way back then to combat her efforts, we have a much stronger bond today. I never knew what to expect from day to day because when Marjory got a wild hair anything could happen. It just didn't work having someone on the outside running our lives.

Chapter Nineteen

When I was pregnant with my first child I was very afraid that Pete would do something crazy, like force me to have an abortion. He had proven in the past that he often made decisions for me with little or no information. He never would ask me what I wanted or thought about my own situation. If he had decided to force me to have an abortion, I would not have been able to prevent it. He had complete legal authority over my person and my property. It was my body right? Actually, in this case, my body was Pete's to do with as he pleased. This situation made me very uncomfortable. I didn't really know Pete or what he might be capable of doing. Before he became my guardian, Pete had only been my mother's lawyer and friend.

During this time he made noises about some kind of training for me on how to be a mother. I have discovered though that parenthood is something that comes naturally, it can't be taught. I never did receive parenting classes like Pete wanted.

He underestimated me though, as usual. I had my baby and am a fine mother.

Actually, today I have two sons.

When I was pregnant with my first son, I asked Pete for some of my money so I could go buy baby essentials in preparation for his arrival. He insisted that Randi and I give him an itemized budget. We had to list each item we wanted for the baby and then call multiple stores here in town to find out how much money each item was going to cost. Then we had to submit this budget to Pete for his approval before he would release any of my money for the supplies. He made me do this all the time when I would ask for money for anything; if he was inclined to give it to me. He really seemed to like the power trip he had over me.

While I was pregnant with my first son I experienced something very interesting. As I said earlier, I had been experiencing a higher than normal sex drive since the tumor. When I became pregnant, my drive was very much enhanced. After I gave birth though my drive dropped to normal levels and has never sky rocketed since. It was as if when I gave birth, along with my body being relieved of my child and the afterbirth products, the abnormally high sex drive was also sloughed off.

I find this very interesting. Perhaps this knowledge could in some way assist other people who have experienced this after a brain injury.

I was not concerned about how I would take care of my baby with my limited vision. I had experience caring for children prior to my blindness and I knew many tricks on how to modify things to make them work for me.

When my son was born I found that I took to motherhood like a duck to water. My son was 11 pounds, 4 ounces and 24 inches long when he was born so he certainly wasn't a delicate little creature. This helped me with any anxiety I may have felt.

God played a funny joke on me, a blind mother, by giving me a baby with a built-in squirt gun. I quickly learned how to protect myself from him. Because of my limited vision I was extra careful to get his diapers on him just right. This made the process of diapering him take longer so I couldn't hurry to cover him up. I developed the habit of leaving a "pee towel" on the changing table. I found that hand towels worked perfect for covering him so he wouldn't aim at me.

My son had such an appetite, I couldn't breast feed him for long after he was born. I switched to formula. I found that having a group of "baa baas" in the cupboard with liners and dry formula in them, waiting for my son to be hungry, worked well. When I had a break from caring for him, I would wash up dirty bottles, place new liners in them and measure the appropriate amount of dry formula into them. I would then stick them in the "baa baa cupboard" until he was hungry. Then my husband or I could run, grab one, and add warm water to it and give it to my baby. When he was hungry, he certainly made it known so it was nicer to get him fed quickly.

My son was very advanced. He took his first steps at six months and was walking or running everywhere at nine months. This enabled me to get back out on the bus quickly after he was born. I found a baby leash at a local store that I would put around his wrist and I would hold the other end so he couldn't go far if he broke away from me when we were out on the bus together. I could then use my cane in my other hand. Any baby stuff I would need on our outing I would carry in a backpack. My mobility instructor worked with my son and me to make sure we were safe when we traveled together.

When my son would try to sneak stuff from the cupboards at home, he couldn't. He would get frustrated because I could "see" him with the eyes in the back of my head. My hearing is so acute that I always knew what he was getting into just from the noises behind me when I was working around the house. I would say something like "Get out of that... cupboard!" and he would wonder how I knew what he was doing. I told him that I could see him with the eyes on the back of my head. This worked; he didn't know what to make of mommy and her "eyes."

Another strategy that worked well for me was trying to keep my home peaceful when the boys were babies. When the house is peaceful and somewhat quiet, you can hear everything that your children are doing.

I also found that there are many talking and large print devices for blind and low vision people to use that can help in parenting; things like talking thermometers, talking bathroom scales and many other useful tools. When it came to dosing my children with medications when they were sick, the best things I found were chewable vitamins and cold medicines. You can ask your doctor when he is prescribing medicine if it is available in a form that does not require a dropper or a syringe for measuring. There are also these really cool strips now for administering cold medicine to children. If you have to give cold medicine to your child before he can chew up a chewable pill, ask your doctor if you can cut it in half to make the dosage right for him and if so, you can then crush it up and put it in liquid or something soft that he can eat. Like I said, you can find a way.

The most challenging part of parenting as a blind mother has definitely been potty training. How do you explain to a child how to do it? When you have boys, you can't demonstrate it when you are a woman. When you are a blind mother, you can't see your son grab himself or doing the potty dance. I must confess, potty training was the one area where I felt totally inadequate. I worked with my son for several weeks with no real progress. Then my step daughter stayed home sick from school one day. She saw my son grab himself. She hustled him into the bathroom and put him on the potty. Then he got it! My older son helped with potty training my second son.

The most important tip I could give someone when it comes to blind parenting is to keep the baby things clean and well organized. It cuts down on wasted time and energy and it prevents a lot of frustration. When my boys were babies, I kept extra crib sheets next to the crib. The organization makes it much easier when your baby spits up or his diaper blows out in his crib. It saves time and effort if you can just strip the mattress, wipe it down with a Clorox wipe, and replace it with a clean sheet. You will save yourself lots of stress if the sheet is readily available instead of trying to go wash bed clothes in the middle of the night when your baby is sick. Likewise, having several changes of clothes available for your baby is also helpful.

I have found many tools to help make motherhood more manageable and thus have been able to take good care of my children. The early years are the most important when it comes to safety. I was able to work through the challenges and so can other blind parents. I hope no one allows their disabilities to prevent them from living their lives to the fullest. "Where there's a will, there's a way."

If you are looking for someone to ask about how to live life or do anything as a blind person, don't ask an "expert" in a lab coat, ask someone who has done it.

Chapter Twenty

When Randi and I first got married, my stepson was living with us. After I had my first son, my stepdaughter eventually got mad at her mom and came to live with us also. Actually, for several years, my two stepchildren pretty much took turns. Every six months or so they would trade places, usually because one or both of them got mad at which ever parent they were living with at the time and my husband catered to their whims. My stepson shortly realized that he had it better with us and that we really loved him and wanted him to be safe and happy. He decided he would rather live with us and follow our rules. My stepdaughter continued to bounce around and be unstable though.

During those early years of our marriage there was a lot of stress. Stress between my stepdaughter and me, stress between my stepson and his dad, stress brought into our home by Marjory and her friends she had working in my home, and stress created by Pete. From this throne in Havre, he felt qualified to insert himself into our situation in Missoula. Due to his lack of knowledge about the situation, his actions created even greater problems for us. Having him in complete control of my life created so much havoc for me.

When Randi and I got married, Pete insisted on taking over the responsibility of paying our family's medical bills. Of course, this was a mistake. It enabled Pete to screw with us and make our lives even more stressful. He simply stopped paying the bills several times. Pete seemed to be confused by the bills when they would show that the insurance had

paid zero dollars on a bill. He didn't understand that there was a deduct-
ible that had to be met. When this happened, he would call me up in his
confusion full of anger and hostility. He would accuse me and/or Randi
of trying to pull something; of trying to get additional funds from my
trust. I really hated having to defend my husband to my guardian all of
the time. Pete was so busy trying to protect my money *from* me that he
failed to do his job: protect *me*.

Pete was such a bully. He was used to pushing me around because I
let him get away with it. After I got married, he tried to bully my husband
also. He tried to trample my husband's parental rights. My husband put
his foot down and told Pete in no uncertain terms that he (Pete) was not
going to make decisions for our children. I was not certain what rights
I had maintained after Pete had been appointed guardian so I couldn't
exercise any to protect my children.

Pete used his power as guardian to obtain private medical information on my husband and our children. He completely violated the
HIPPA laws. He had a legal right to my medical records as my guardian but he did not have rights to Randi's or our children's records. He
took information from our children's records and twisted it to make our
situation seem totally dysfunctional. For example, he accused my step
daughter of having been tested for methamphetamine use when the bill
was actually for an allergy test. He always presented his accusations as
"fact" not to be questioned. It was so difficult for me, trying to explain to
him what was actually going on in the face of his ire all the time. Since
we were just a normal family, he had to trump up charges against us
that weren't true.

It was during these early years of our marriage that Joanne made
another attempt to regain control of my money. She knew I was having
a lot of problems with Pete. She also knew that I loved my stepfather
very much. She applied a lot of pressure to me, trying to convince me to
fire Pete and have her husband, my stepfather, appointed as my guardian. During this time my mom had been cheating on my dad and he was
trying to win her love back from whence it had gone. Who knows what

my stepfather might have done to make her happy if he had been given control of my assets. She really thought I was an idiot. That would have put me back under her thumb completely.

Even though Pete was her friend, it wasn't very often when I saw him making decisions that benefited Joanne rather than me. He usually tried to do what he thought was best for me. Unfortunately, his decisions tended to be harmful to me due to his lack of first-hand knowledge of my situation.

Talk about no honor amongst thieves. Joanne had her friend, Pete, appointed in order to keep control of my money. When she saw a chance to snatch control from him, however, she grabbed for it. It's quite funny now, all these years later, to think about it.

Pete's problem was that he never consulted with me regarding my own situation. He had a very suspicious nature and only listened to other people talking about what *they* thought should happen in my life. I was treated with suspicion and contempt, as if I were a danger to myself. Pete never should have allowed himself to be appointed to the guardianship. He was far from a neutral party without interest in my assets. Havre was also too far away for him to function in that capacity the way he should have. The court should not have appointed him to that position either. I wish the court would have done a little research into the background of my situation before the judge made his ruling.

This chaotic nightmare went on for a long time. Then I asked Pete for some of my money. Usually, when I would ask Pete for money (any amount over the fixed income he had me living on) he would become enraged as if I were out of line, then demand a meeting with Marjory. As a result, we would periodically have meetings. They were called "team meetings." The team usually consisted of Pete, Marjory, Dr. Johnson, my Mom and step Dad and myself. After I got married my husband was also part of the "team."

These were bitch out sessions. They would debate how much of a screw up I was. After I got married, it became about what screw ups Randi and I both were. Back then I was expected to walk a fine line, not making any bad decisions. If I made a decision that was viewed by anyone on the "team" as a "bad" decision, that would bring down the wrath upon my family and me.

This abuse went on for years. I was unable to think fast enough to keep ahead of the barrage of criticism that was lodged at us in those meetings. Anything Randi or I would say was quickly dismissed as unimportant or irrelevant. These people were highly educated and had an agenda of their own to fulfill.

I am good at expressing myself in writing, when I have time to contemplate my words, but I couldn't keep up with these professional people who had spent their careers discussing these issues.

I was also very affected by the negative words I had always heard from these people who should have lifted me up instead of tearing me down.

Chapter Twenty-One

*A*t one point, I called Pete and asked for some of my money. He became angry and threatened to take me to court to have a "review of spending" before the judge here in Missoula. I panicked, not because Randi or I had anything to hide but because I knew what would happen in court. I would have no representation and neither would Randi. We would be going head to head with Pete, who was completely ignorant about what was going on here. In his camp was Marjory, who always twisted the facts to fit her agenda.

I was in great anguish. This could mean real problems for my marriage and my baby. Pete was capable of anything.

I fell on my knees and asked the Lord for some direction. I felt impressed to call my pastor. When I met with my pastor and told him what was going on, he recommended a lawyer he knew.

Because Pete had me on a fixed income I could only afford to give the lawyer a $200 retainer. I told the lawyer the whole sordid affair. He announced it was clear that I was not "incapacitated" so we would simply challenge the guardianship.

This shocked me. I didn't really know what the word "incapacitated" meant although I certainly knew how it had impacted my life. I was thrilled at the prospect of having it removed.

I hired the attorney. Over time he decided he didn't have enough court room experience to handle my case by himself. This was when Bruce, another attorney, was brought on board. Once Bruce joined the team, Pete decided that the only reason we needed two lawyers was so one could represent Randi and the other, me. He made the allegation that I was being forced to pay for an attorney for Randi. Yet again, another crazy accusation from Pete.

Bruce and I had a lot of discussions that year I was in litigation with Pete. I learned a lot from Bruce about how guardianships should be handled.

During that year Pete behaved true to form. He acted angry and hostile toward us like never before. He behaved rather paranoid. He had accused me of misappropriating my own funds in the past. It was very strange the way he acted about giving up control over me and my funds. I began to suspect that he himself may in fact be guilty of some misdeeds with my legal or financial affairs.

When I filed the petition to fire Pete, I changed my phone number so he couldn't call and threaten me. He attempted to talk the judge into forcing me to give him my new phone number. Once again he underestimated me. I had saved a threatening message from him that he had left on my voicemail. When I found out what he was trying to do I gave a copy of it to my attorney so he could play it for the judge. I wanted the judge to hear an example of the verbal abuse I had always suffered at Pete's hands. Thankfully the judge then decided not to force me to give Pete my new phone number. Having my attorney to run interference between Pete and me was wonderful. For that whole year, I didn't have to live in fear of Pete's wrath.

While we were in litigation with Pete, he insisted I undergo yet another neuropsychological evaluation with Dr. Johnson. This was always his answer when I was trying to achieve something he didn't want me to do, i.e. marrying Randi. A complete neuropsychological evaluation consists of many tests that look at several different facets of how the brain functions.

My attorney advised me that I had to submit to the testing so I called and made the appointment with Dr. Johnson. When I arrived for the exam I underwent two brief tests. He then told me to leave and he would call me to schedule more testing later.

I never heard back from him.

Several days after the deadline for discovery, set by the judge, had come and gone my lawyer heard from Pete's attorney. Dr. Johnson wanted to do more tests. My attorney advised me that I didn't have to submit to these tests because they had messed around and missed the deadline set by the judge.

When I filed my petition to fire Pete, he hired a lawyer here in Missoula to represent him while he fought me on my petition. The bank also hired a lawyer to represent them and fight me in my endeavors to regain my civil rights and property.

The judge imposed sanctions on me. He forced me to pay not only my attorneys but also the attorneys for Pete and the bank. I was also forced to continue to pay Pete his monthly salary for being my "guardian", even though during that year I could not have any contact with him because we were in litigation. I was also forced to pay the costs for Pete and the bank so they could fight me. I have strong feelings about how much power judges have over innocent people. It so easily goes awry. I felt like the judge was punishing me for daring to challenge the guardianship and attempting to regain my civil rights and property.

I had become aware prior to filing my petition that the judge was also friends with Pete. I had arrived at the court for an anticipated hearing before the judge. The judge was seated up at his bench when Pete walked into the courtroom. The judge actually called out to Pete from up on his bench! He exclaimed "Pete!" as if greeting an old friend. I shuddered to realize the connection. This told me in no uncertain terms that the judge knew Pete and appeared to like him. The deck was stacked against me from the very beginning.

While I was in litigation with Pete that year I had to go to the court house and get some documents on my case. They were sealed documents. Since they were sealed I figured they were the documents pertaining to the original settlement. These documents were sealed for my protection all those years ago.

When I went to get the documents that day I was so affected by stress that I thought I would become physically ill. I had a horrible headache and couldn't stop shaking. I was all by myself and I had to go to the clerk's office and request the sealed documents.

After she found them and ran copies for me I quickly left.

When I got home with the documents and read them with my husband I was horrified to learn that the guardianship had been instigated by my four "loving" parents. The hell that my life had become was created by the four people who should have loved and supported me. They had tried to hide the truth and bury their actions by having it all sealed by a judge.

The documents were letters that were written by my parents in 1997. It was clear from the letters that my parents had made a lot of assumptions way back then about what was really going on with me. Once again, no one had discussed anything with me.

It was years later when I had the opportunity to discuss these letters with my stepmother. In an effort to defend their actions she blurted out "We had to protect the money!" That was when I told her I had lost my civil rights because of what they had done to me. Her confession was also very revealing because she and my biological dad had always given me a song and dance about how they didn't care about the money, they just wanted what was best for me. Fat chance!

Chapter Twenty-Two

When the date arrived for the court hearing regarding my 'incapacitation', pandemonium ensued. The proceedings were ridiculous! Dr. Johnson's testimony proved him to be inept and incompetent. Marjory presented hear-say evidence that only proved she did not have my best interests at heart. The financial "experts" were completely inaccurate regarding my funds. All in all, Pete's case was a complete sham.

When Dr. Johnson was on the witness stand under cross examination by my attorney, I found out why I had always felt so horrible when he was treating me. He didn't even know what part of my brain was damaged! He had been treating me for the wrong type of brain injury all those years! Pete had relied on his opinion for years and he didn't even know what was going on with me. At this point I began to understand why Pete always misjudged my situation. I wish Pete had simply asked me.

When Marjory was on the witness stand she conducted herself true to form. She made completely false accusations toward my husband and step children. She made our home life sound like a circus. At times it was like a circus due to the chaos created by Marjory and her friends. Our actual family life was rather normal. Sure we had some issues, but they were just normal issues when dealing with teenagers and step parents. She made it sound like my husband beat me in an effort to keep me subservient to him. Her testimony made it sound like my step children were doing drugs in my living room and all manner of other illicit activities. She made me out to be a severely brain damaged, helpless invalid whose husband and step children were taking advantage of her. The judge also allowed Marjory to present hear-say evidence about statements allegedly made to her by her friends who were working in my home. These 'friends' never did testify.

A woman who worked for the bank in Minneapolis also flew out to Missoula to testify against me. She had never even met me and could not contribute any firsthand knowledge of the situation.

Pete also hired a financial person to evaluate my assets and make a judgment call concerning whether or not my account would be able to survive long term at the current rate of spending. Of course according to him it could not. No one pointed out that I was living on a fixed income and the lion's share of the money coming out of my account was being spent to support Pete's guardianship, since he was not available to be here in Missoula.

As it ultimately turned out the financial guy Pete had hired was totally incorrect with his figures. He had completely left out a large part of my assets in his figures. This was not known at the time though.

Another person who testified against me was Dr. Web. She was a psychologist who saw me before I was under the guardianship. I had always liked and respected Dr. Web, but I feel her testimony should have been rendered invalid because she hadn't seen me since August of 1996, six months prior to me entering the Bridges program. As I pointed out earlier; Bridges was the turning point in my recovery. She was testifying based on old knowledge that was long since irrelevant.

I had to pay for all of this "expert" testimony.

Strangely, in March of 1997 when I was railroaded into the guardianship, no expert testimony was required. Now, when attempting to overturn the guardianship, I had to spend tens of thousands of dollars on "expert" testimony. I had to pay not only my supporting experts, but also those in opposition to me.

The judge somehow missed that Dr. Johnson and Dr. Web had no way of knowing what they were talking about. Marjory convinced him that Randi was abusing me and my step children were doing drugs.

Marjory also testified that my little boy, who wasn't quite two years old yet, was intentionally a naughty boy. She went on to say that my son did this to be more difficult for me. What a kangaroo court! Not only were these accusations untrue, but they had nothing to do with whether or not I was incapacitated. Dr. Johnson and Marjory were the only ones who were really in a position to know what was going on and both were inept.

I had undergone a complete neuropsychological evaluation with Dr. Paulson, another neuropsychologist in the community. His findings were that I was completely competent to handle my affairs. Of course this opinion was at odds with what Pete was trying to accomplish; keeping his guardianship in place.

Ultimately the judge was more concerned about my physical safety and protecting the damn money than whether or not I was indeed incapacitated. The judge didn't ask me anything regarding these issues that day in court.

When the judge made his ruling I went into shock, into a type of auto pilot. I remember interrupting the judge as he was ruling against me. I told him I would submit to the continuation of the guardianship but I wanted a local guardian who could really get to know my family and learn what was going on in my home. I also told him I wanted my trust moved to Missoula. This way, I could learn how to manage my money and hopefully someday become free of the guardianship. When Pete had brought me to Missoula in 1997 he had intentionally left my trust in Minneapolis so I couldn't have any contact with my trust officer. This prevented me from gaining any real knowledge of how my trust worked.

I also told the judge that I didn't need a case manager so Marjory was fired. I really wish I could have been the one to make that phone call.

Pete's guardianship had been allowed to carry on for seven years.

After the hearing in January of 2004, I obtained a document that discussed the legal definition of "incapacitated." The definition is incredibly vague, thus allowing judges and attorneys to interpret it however they want. I think this term needs to be better defined in order to prevent this from happening to any other innocent people.

Another document I was able to obtain after court was a copy of The Bill of Rights.

As I read through this most important portion of our Constitution, I was shocked and sickened to discover that Pete, Joanne and all their cronies had violated my civil rights. They had denied me the rights guaranteed to me in the first, third, fourth, fifth and sixth amendments. As a result of this miscarriage of justice, my second amendment rights will always be denied me unless I can somehow convince another judge to restore them to me.

You may be asking yourself, why would a blind woman need a firearm? That is not the point. All Americans are guaranteed this right, not just those who can see clearly and I am actually able to hunt with the assistance of my husband.

There are special exceptions to this amendment such as violent criminals, who do not have this right any longer, but I committed no such crime. The court just decided to deny me my civil rights.

Keep in mind that this also means I cannot carry a concealed weapon for my own protection either. I cannot carry a hand gun, a knife or even a bottle of mace in my purse to protect myself if I am mugged, raped or molested in any other way.

Worst of all, the state of Montana allowed them to do this to me.

That day in court when the judge denied my petition, he refused to make a ruling on whether or not I was indeed "incapacitated." When I got out of court I sought help from the ADA (American Disabilities Act) to help me make this all right but they flat refused to even look at my case once they found out that I was under a guardianship. Even the ADA was too weak to fight back against a power such as this.

Part Five

A New Beginning

Chapter Twenty-Three

After I got out of court in 2004, when the judge had ruled against me, I needed a new guardian. Bruce introduced me to a lawyer he knew in town who actually had experience handling guardianships; unlike Pete.

When I met Vern I was still quite emotionally traumatized after my experiences in court. I felt like I had once again been railroaded by another judge. I was very uncomfortable about Vern because I had such horrible experiences with Pete. As it turned out though, Vern was a completely different guardian.

During the course of his guardianship, several situations arose that enabled me to get to know Vern. I came to know and trust him in a way I never had Pete.

The first was when I needed to hire someone to work in my home, driving for me and assisting with household activities.

In the past, whenever I made any decision, I had to clear it with Pete or Marjory first so when I needed to hire someone, I called Vern to seek his permission. His response was, "Do you need a case manager to get this done for you?"

This startled me; he was allowing me to do it for myself.

Later, I called Vern to ask for some of my money. His response was, "It's your money."

Wow, imagine this after living with the hostility and craziness of Pete and his cronies for so many years!

Vern was an anomaly. I had met so many lawyers over the years since my mom had initially filed her lawsuit and Vern was one of a kind. He sincerely cared about what was best for my family, not just his pocketbook. Even though his hourly rate was substantially higher than Pete's, my guardianship costs were a fraction of what they had once been.

Vern was much more reasonable than Pete had ever been but it took a long time before I could call and discuss any issue with him without experiencing a great deal of stress. When I would have to call him I would shake, experience headaches, and feel nauseous. I started to realize at this point that I had suffered a lot more abuse at the hands of Pete and Marjory than I had realized. I should not have had this reaction when I thought about calling Vern. I was very angry that I had been so mistreated.

During Vern's guardianship we didn't have a single "team" meeting. It was amazing! Since he was right there in Missoula, he was able to do his job without the assistance of all those extra people. When Pete had been guardian, it was clearly a case of too many Chiefs and not enough Indians. My life was much more enjoyable under Vern's guardianship than it had ever been under Pete's. I had unobstructed one on one contact with Vern, no case manager running interference for him. It was like a breath of fresh air.

One instance of Vern's support was when I began experiencing flashbacks involving Joanne. I first discussed these memories with my husband. He told me that what I was remembering was my mom molesting me. This was initially difficult for me to accept. After further thought, I realized if my teacher, bus driver or anyone else had done what she did, I would have recognized it as "molestation". Because it was my mom, I figured it must be okay. I know she did the same thing to at least one of my little sisters and I suspect she did it to all four of us. Needless to say, I don't allow my mom near my children.

I discussed these memories with Vern. He instructed me to write down what I was remembering. After I recorded my experience, I returned it to Vern for his records. There needed to be documentation of the incidents.

When we got out of court, the bank found a local trust officer for my account. The guy was a jerk to me and talked down to me all the time. This wasn't just my opinion, my husband and my sister also felt this way. I was embarrassed when he would come to my house to meet with me. He was very arrogant and I didn't care for the attitude he used when he was in my home. It was rather creepy the way he would speak to my children also.

On one occasion he came to my house. While here, he shared with me some personal problems he was having. He told me that as a result of these problems he was moving out of town. When he left town I no longer had a local trust officer, as the judge had ordered. The bank deceived the judge on this fact by using a P.O. box in Missoula on the forms they would file with the court each year when it was time for the annual accounting. I don't think the judge ever found out that the bank was pulling the wool over his eyes.

During the years Vern served as my guardian there were a lot of changes in my life.

I gave birth to my second son in 2006. When he was born he stopped breathing. The doctors weren't sure if he would survive. I remember during this time feeling the old suffocating grief on my chest again. I was in despair, how could I help my child? I think I understand what my mom went through so many years ago a little better now. When I was finally able to hold my child, I was at the hospital every night to rock him to sleep and place him in his crib in the NICU (Neonatal Intensive Care Unit). Prior to that, I was there every available minute; holding his little hand, praying for, and cooing to him. It was so difficult. I could talk to him but he couldn't even whimper in response because he had a respirator hose down his throat and I couldn't see him. All I could do was hold his hand and gently feel around on his body, being careful not to mess up the tubes and tape all over his little form. Because of my limited vision, my world is a tactile one. I couldn't be certain of anything regarding my child's condition until I was able to hold him. Until then, it was like being lost in a dark void, searching for some kind of hope for the survival of my son. He was in the NICU for fifteen days following his birth and I couldn't even hold him until he was seven days old.

As a result of not having oxygen when he was born, he exhibits some difficulties but he is gradually getting better.

If he had been born when Pete was guardian I shudder to think what probably would have happened. Vern, as usual, was very supportive of us during this time. I really appreciated the way Vern conducted himself while we were going through this difficult time in our family. He let me know that he would be there if we needed him, but would otherwise stay in the background.

While under Vern's guardianship, life went on for all of us like any other independent family. In 2009 my husband had open heart surgery in Rochester, Minnesota. My step kids both grew up and moved out on their own. Both of my sons also started school during this period of time.

I also began to travel independently outside of my general community. My husband is the one who encouraged me to do this. I now travel anywhere and anytime I get the opportunity.

During my travels I have had many interactions with the TSA (Transportation Safety Administration). Not all of these experiences were positive. There have been times where I have approached the TSA area and had my white cane ripped from my hand. I was then nudged toward the metal detector. On one occasion, after they took my cane from me, they gave me an inferior cane that was actually a support cane. It was much too short to use for obstacle detection.

I am usually the one who is selected for the "random" search. As if a terrorist would pose as a blind person to attempt to trick the TSA! My worst experience with the TSA was the time I was traveling alone with my children. They took me by the arm and started dragging me away to an unknown location. I had to quickly instruct my older son to stay where he was and keep his little brother with him; I would be right back (I hoped). I honestly had no idea where they were taking me and when, or even if, I would be back.

I have found that the worst problem at TSA, when dealing with blind people, is the lack of communication. TSA agents do not communicate with me when I am there going through the process; so I have taken it upon myself to communicate with them. When I first approach the TSA area, I surrender my cane to them so they can put it through the metal detector. I then extend my arms out in front of me, so they can guide me through the walk-through metal detector with their arms extended from the other side. This works well. They then guide me to a seat where I can put my shoes back on and retrieve my items from the conveyor belt. I really wish the TSA would be trained to interact with blind people more appropriately.

I never had these experiences with traveling before. When Pete had been in control, I was not allowed to leave town without his permission.

Once I began traveling, I found that I loved getting out of Missoula. We had all experienced such treachery from Marjory, Pete and their friends, it was liberating to get away and discover that there was a better world out there.

When I got out of court in 2004, I experienced so many different emotions. I remember I didn't feel safe in my own home. I purchased a security system for my home. I also took down my flimsy curtains from my large picture window on the front of my house and put up heavy drapes so people couldn't see in.

I also didn't feel safe traveling around town anymore. I couldn't be sure who might be lurking around, watching me. Marjory and her friends all lived here and I also heard from a reliable source that Pete had moved to the area. I have run into Marjory and several of her friends on multiple occasions. These people participated in the conspiracy against my family and I just don't feel safe here anymore.

I have been involved in three car accidents since I moved to Missoula in 1997. As a result of all these car accidents, I experience a great amount of pain in my neck and back during the cold winters here.

I would prefer to live in a warmer climate. We are currently looking in Arizona for a new home. There are many things making it difficult for us to move. I really don't like living here anymore but my children are in a good school and Pete had forced me to buy a house here. It is very difficult to relocate your entire family when you own property in a community. The home we are looking for in Arizona would be our primary residence, but I would keep the house in Missoula for us to visit in the summers.

In 2011 I again filed a petition with the court to terminate the guardianship.

It was almost a year from the time I filed my petition until the hearing actually occurred. During this year I again experienced symptoms of too much stress. I had horrible headaches. I shook uncontrollably and nearly became physically ill when I thought about the impending court date.

This time was different though. The guardian and the conservator both took a neutral stance if not an outright supportive position on my petition.

In court the judge ruled in my favor on my petition. The turning point seemed to occur when my attorney pointed out that my civil rights had been violated by the administration of the guardianship.

It is really sad the way this was done to me in the name of protecting the money and no one considered that my rights were being violated until I pointed it out. Isn't this the U.S. of A. anymore?

At this point it has been over a year since I got out of court. These past months have been very difficult for me. I have had to deal with a great amount of anger at the way 15 years of my life were lost. I am angry at the stolen choices and missed opportunities. I can't help but wonder what may have turned out differently had Pete's guardianship been handled properly. My life may have turned out drastically different had my mother allowed me to get treatment for my brain injury many years earlier. I think that someone should have been overseeing her treatment of me much closer when I was young. Coming to terms with the devastating loss of so many years has been incredibly difficult for me. How does a person go on after something like this? Only God has the answers.

All I can do is chalk it all up to His will and look for the positives in it. There are many positives that have resulted from this miscarriage of justice. I have two beautiful sons. I also have a dear friend in Vern. I have grown a lot through these experiences. I met and married my best friend.

I have learned there are facilities in this country that a blind person can attend to learn braille and other skills of daily living. These skills are far more intensive than those I was taught through the Visual Services all those years ago.

Currently it is my goal to attend one of these facilities so I can learn braille and acquire those skills I missed out on. Once I learn these additional skills, my family's quality of life will be greatly enhanced from where it is today.

There are many difficult situations I describe in my book. I can definitely see God's hand in all of it, however. If it hadn't been for the initial traumatic brain injury, I never would have come to Missoula to enter the Community Bridges Program. It was here in Missoula that God has brought Randi into my life. He is now my best friend. God's gift of my two sons complete my life. Although the experience in court in 1997 was difficult, I can see how God's hand moved Pete to bring me to Missoula. Frankly, even though there were many years of struggle to deal with some very hard situations, I am convinced that all these things were in God's timing. Someday I will surely know how even the scars I still carry will be worked together for my good. In a way, it is exciting to imagine what God has in store for me.

This is the end of my story but the beginning of my future.

Part 6

Closing Thoughts

I have written this book for multiple reasons.

I want to bring to the attention of the legal system that the laws pertaining to guardianships must be changed.

I want to help families and individuals whose lives have been impacted by a TBI to be better equipped to deal with the massive life changes.

If you are looking for more information regarding blindness for yourself or a loved one, I strongly encourage you to contact the National Federation of the Blind (NFB). The national headquarters for the NFB is located in Baltimore, Maryland but each state has an affiliate. Each affiliate is comprised of different chapters located throughout its' respective state. If only my parents had known to contact the NFB when I was a child, I could have received the training I so desperately needed much earlier in life.

I also want to give medical professionals a clear picture of what a person with a TBI experiences during various stages of their recovery.

I want to make people aware of what their rights are because if we don't know what they are, they can so easily be taken from us.

If I can prevent even one person from having to experience what I have had to go through, then this has all been worth it.

Author's Note

his book is utterly true. I have changed or intentionally omitted the names of individuals to protect the innocent and the guilty. Any resemblance to actual individuals living or dead is purely coincidental.

While writing this book, it became necessary for me to dig up some old records. I have never bothered to look up these old records because I wasn't sure if they were still available and I also wasn't sure if I truly wanted to know what happened way back when my story began. As I said in my story, I have never consciously remembered what transpired later that last day before I went blind.

When I finally broke down and sought out the old files, after much difficulty in trying to locate them, I found them at long last.

What I learned in the files was bitter sweet. On that last day when my mom took me to see Dr. Andrews, he performed a lumbar puncture on me and ultimately put me in the hospital in Chester. I was there over night. Throughout the night, as my condition deteriorated, Dr. Andrews only prescribed various pain medications and anti-nausea medicine. The files indicate that at one point I was so close to death I only responded to pain stimuli; nothing else. The next day he finally decided to call the ambulance from Great Falls to come. As a result of the pressure from the tumor and the spinal tap (which was also an act of malpractice because it greatly increased the pressure in my head) according to several expert's reports I read in the files, my brain herniated causing my death. More than one expert stated that Dr. Andrews "failed to provide the standard of care" that would be expected in these circumstances. My mother witnessed my death in the ambulance. I can now understand a little better how my mom is able to "act" like I'm dead because she actually watched it happen. I believe that when I wound up surviving, it was that much harder for her to relax and expect that I would actually live. Thus, it was easier for her to disconnect herself from me. The money offered her some comfort from her grief. She never could accept that I am her daughter because I am so different from the daughter she once knew and I died, after all. Why not pretend I'm still dead and protect herself from hurting like that again? I'm not a trained doctor but that makes some sense to me at least and like I said in my book, I've struggled with the rift in our relationship for so long. I lost a lot more that day in April of 1989 than just my vision. I have lost all these years of liberty, I have lost my relationship with most of my family and I have lost much of my intellectual ability. Like I've already said though, God will work it all together for my good. I just need to wait on His timing.

An important aspect of my personal beliefs is that God *does* answer all of our prayers. Sometimes, the answer is yes. Other times the answer is no. Many times, God tells us to wait on His timing.

About the Author

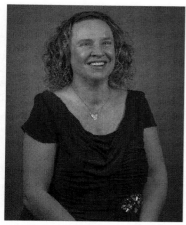

Rebecca S Meadows lives in Missoula, Montana with her husband and her two children. She finds purpose in life while caring for her family. She is devoted to making sure her children are happy and healthy while also making sure they get a good education. She also travels extensively and enjoys meeting new people while having new experiences. She is a proud member of the NFB. She is very passionate about her faith and she strongly believes in the rights of individual Americans. She considers herself somewhat of an expert in living with a TBI such as hers. She has, after all, been living with hers for over 24 years. She doubtless has much to offer that can never be taught in an institution of higher learning. It is her goal to make sure the rights of disabled citizens are protected. She believes the best way to do this is to educate as many people as she can about what our rights are. She wants to prevent what happened to her from happening to any other innocent people. She wants to help other disabled Americans understand that there is a place for them in our society.

Photo by: The Real McCoy Photography